MEDICAL MAVERICKS

VOLUME TWO

N.A.
2018-2019

HUGH DESAIX RIORDAN, M.D.

Bio-Communications Press
3100 North Hillside
Wichita, Kansas 67219 USA

MEDICAL MAVERICKS
Volume Two

BIO-COMMUNICATIONS PRESS
3100 North Hillside Avenue
Wichita, Kansas 67219 USA

ISBN 0-942333-09-8
Library of Congress Catalog Card Number: 88-63321

First Edition

Published in The United States of America

cover drawing by Moore Anderson

BCP and Bio-Communications Press are service marks of
The Olive W. Garvey Center
for the Improvement of Human Functioning, Inc.

"MEDICAL HISTORY involves social and economic as well as biological content and presents one of the central themes of human experience."

RICHARD H. SKYROCK

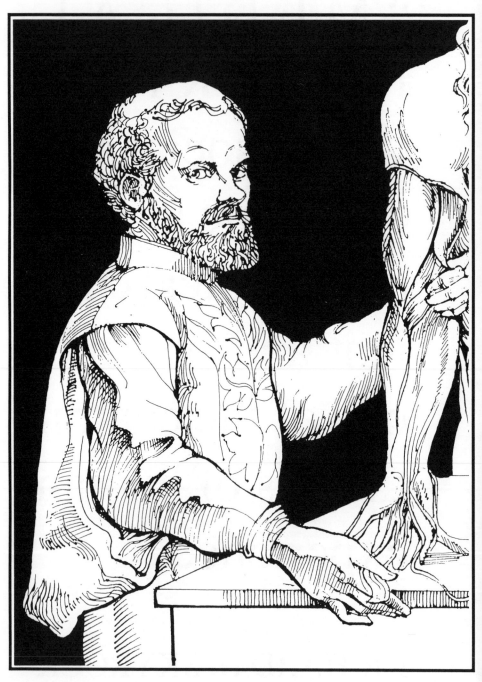

VESALIUS

TABLE OF CONTENTS

MAVERICK

The word maverick is derived from an American pioneer, Samuel A. Maverick, who chose to not brand his cattle. Through usage the word maverick, in addition to meaning an unbranded range animal, has come to mean an independent individual who refuses to conform to his/her group.

This book is about such independent individuals who followed the advice found in this anonymous quotation.

Do not follow where

The path may lead

Go instead where

There is no path

And leave a trail

DEDICATION

This book, like its predecessor, is dedicated to the memory of all those medical doctors who, since history has been recorded, have contributed to the progress of the science and art of medicine.

This book is also dedicated to the countless numbers of those people we call patients who have, through the ages, endured much, suffered greatly and benefited considerably from those who have practiced the science and art of medicine.

This book is dedicated to the maverick in you—that wonderful element perhaps obvious, perhaps hidden which moved you to choose to read this bit of writing.

Lastly, this book is dedicated to Olive White Garvey. Her ninety-six years of active participation in life have allowed her to develop an in-depth understanding and appreciation for the maverick spirit which she, too, embodies.

H.D.R.

ACKNOWLEDGEMENTS

Little did I realize prior to the release of *Medical Mavericks,* Volume One how enormously satisfying the feedback would be from so many of you who graciously provided me with your impressions of the work.

Your comments have truly inspired me not only to release Volume Two a little early but also to accelerate my efforts on Volume Three.

This second volume of the planned trilogy has come to fruition following arduous research, dedicated input and skillful editing by Jeanne Johnston and Rebecca Burke.

The final production of this volume has been made possible by the fine efforts of Barbara Nichols of Bio-Communications Press, Teresa Riordan who performed final editing and Moore Anderson whose sketch of Vesalius appears on the cover.

Many thanks to you who made comments such as "I don't know when I have enjoyed a volume as much as I have *Medical Mavericks.* Please hurry along with Volume II. I shall be eagerly awaiting it."

H. D. R.

FOREWORD

Whether it is the most ancient Cardano or the more recent Wright the vignettes repeatedly reflect the wisdom of Schopenhauer's observation that new thought and new truths most often go through three stages. First they are ridiculed. Next they are violently opposed. Then, finally they are accepted as being self-evident.

H. D. R.

CARDANO

"The things which give most reputation to a physician nowadays are his manners, servants, carriage, clothes, smartness, and caginess, all displayed in a sort of artificial and insipid way; learning and experience seem to count for nothing."[1]

Gerolamo Cardano

Gerolamo Cardano (1501-1576), illegitimate son to Chiara Alberio and Fazio Cardano, learned to fend for himself early in life. This independence and determination helped him support himself as he attended university to prepare for medical training. Because of a broad knowledge in philosophy, mathematics, astronomy, and dialectics, he found many young pupils to tutor. Cardano, also an astrologist, cast numerous horoscopes for willing buyers. His skill at dice also won him much needed money because he was able to calculate his risks. In fact, his study of the subject led to the laws of probability as we know them today. He was soon recognized as a brilliant young man. But Cardano had a laconic, caustic manner that made him many enemies. This almost destroyed his chances to earn his doctorate in medicine. The granting of this degree depended upon social qualification as well as upon proof of ability. Three votes had to be cast before the faculty of Padua University finally decided to grant him his degree.

Cardano then set out to Milan to establish a practice there through the College of Physicians. But ill-wishers who had heard of his tactless manner and read his criticism of traditional medicine in On the Differing Opinions of Physicians prohibited his acceptance by enforcing a college statute requiring legitimacy of birth, although exceptions to this statute had often been made before. This was the start of a lifetime of professional difficulties. Moving to small villages and then again to Milan, for the second time refused by the Milanese

1

doctors, his wife miscarrying with each move, Cardano finally settled in Gallarate where he was employed as a ghostwriter by a young nobelman, Filippo Archinto. These years of wandering from town to town, living in destitution, practicing medicine secretly, and enduring the disdain of the Milanese physicians affected Cardano's behavior. He gave the impression of having an unbalanced mind with his self-pitying outpourings to anyone who would listen. He vowed he heard voices haunting him throughout the day and the night. And he claimed that his horoscope predicted imminent death. But in Gallarate the clean mountain air and the distance from his enemies cleared his thinking. This comfortable arrangement dissolved, however, when a campaign against Charles V deprived Cardano of his patron's support. Once again the young couple was destitute. The next spring Cardano's wife Lucia gave birth to a son, Giovanni, a weak baby deformed by a slight spine curvature and the joining of two toes on one foot.

Cardano again decided to travel to Milan although he had no money. He and his wife were forced to beg for their food and shelter until they reached the city's almshouse. Fortunately Filippo Archinto returned from service and re-established their former relationship. He also nominated Cardano to a public lectureship that attracted pupils once again. Cardano then set about writing numerous books on the various subjects he was teaching. Unfortunately he rewrote and republished his previous controversial work under the new title, The Bad Practice of Healing Among Modern Doctors. In this book, he pointed out many practices he called medical errors—"the result of the tribal insecurities of men who banded themselves together and showed the world a surface of pomp and learning that satisfactorily concealed from the beholders the depth of ignorance beneath."[2] But he did not proofread and edit the manuscript so that it was published with all its grammatical and factual errors, which gave offended doctors the means to attack him vehemently. Cardano's stricture only reinforced the physicians' antagonism. On the other hand, it delighted the lay public who were at the mercy of physicians and their mysterious poultices and possets.

Therefore, Cardano's fortune continued to improve. A patient he had once treated secretly had been healed and now wished to offer the doctor an appointment. The patient, a prior of a religious order, had been suffering from tuberculoid leprosy. Cardano had observed his lifestyle and then given his prescription of healing. The prior, in his spiritual dedication, had neglected his bodily needs. Cardano counseled him to sleep regular hours, exercise and eat regularly, bathe frequently, and wear comfortable clothing. The healed prior rewarded Cardano's skill by appointing the doctor as official physician of the priory.

Now Cardano no longer needed the College's approval. Patients hurried to see him, hearing of his simple, commonsense cures that did not cost them the usual extravagant sums of money. Cardano was especially famous for his cure for tuberculosis—a disease that no other doctor could heal. Cardano established the idea of the sanatorium; he ordered clean country air, plenty of rest, a nourishing diet, and simple, undemanding interests. Cardano also differentiated between two prevalent diseases, gonorrhea and syphilis, and developed a treatment that cured syphilis with a special ointment containing mercury.

Seeing his success, the Milanese College of Physicians felt compelled to welcome Cardano into their guild. But in the midst of this triumph, Cardano again made an enemy who would later work to destroy him. Tartaglia, a mathematician who knew a complex cubic equation but would not reveal it, gave Cardano the mathematical problem no one but he, Tartaglia, could compute since only he knew the equation. Cardano figured out the rule himself and published it in The Practice of Arithmetic and Simple Mensuration, although he gave Tartaglia the credit for its discovery. This enraged Tartaglia. Thereafter he began to watch Cardano's every action and keep each logged in his notebooks to be brought out at the correct time. He also fashioned stories about Cardano which he whispered to various important people. After Cardano was named Professor of Medicine at Pavia and Rector of the College at Milan, the Pope offered him the post of papal astrologer which Cardano refused. Tartaglia convinced the Pope's emissary that Cardano meant to offend the Pope with his refusal. He also gave the man a copy of Cardano's Life of Christ, which cast a horoscope for Christ, certainly blasphemous. This was also recorded and saved for the proper moment.

Meanwhile, Cardano's fame as a doctor spread far. He was invited by John Hamilton, Archbishop of St. Andrews in Edinburgh, Scotland, to consult with him on his asthma which no doctor could cure. Cardano observed Hamilton for several months after which he prescribed a simple diet, regular exercise, fresh air, and no more feather mattresses. The archbishop recovered and Cardano returned to Milan.

After his return, his three children, always troubled and difficult, began to create serious problems for themselves and their father. Lucia had died several years previously and Cardano was left to parent the children. His daughter Chiara, a licentious young woman, became pregnant with her brother's child. She aborted the child, but in doing so ruined her chances to have other children. For this reason, after an unwise marriage, she was divorced. Chiara later died in an asylum, insane and paralyzed from syphilis. Cardano's eldest son, Giovanni, became constantly involved in crime. When he was blackmailed into marrying a young woman, he poisoned her and was consequently tortured and executed. Cardano's youngest son, Aldo, a vicious and cruel man, became a torturer for the Inquisition after spending several years in and out of prison for his violence.

Cardano's children's deeds threatened Cardano's sanity and destroyed his reputation. He became extremely paranoid as he saw that people were shunning his presence. He left Milan and began to roam from one city to another, always

4

imagining plots to assassinate him. Perhaps some were true. Authorities, avoiding him because of his ruined reputation, sought to sever their relationship with him. Milan exiled him from the state after accusing him of sodomy and incest.

Tartaglia had been waiting for such a turn in fortune. He thwarted Cardano's attempts to find positions with various universities and cities. And after Cardano had lived seven years in extreme poverty, all of his movements carefully watched and recorded, Tartaglia called for Cardano's arrest and trial by the Inquisition. At the trial, all Cardano's misdeeds, unwise statements, and statements out of context, were used against him. Chief among these was his horoscope of Christ. After the trial Cardano was returned to prison where he lay searching his mind for an influential acquaintance who might help him. He remembered Archbishop Hamilton's request to be called upon if there were ever the need. Cardano wrote at once. The Archbishop effected his release with his statement that Cardano was interested in healing man's body, the dwelling-place of God's souls.

Despite this fortunate release, Cardano was deprived of what he considered worthwhile. He could no longer lecture publicly or publish his books. A devoted pupil, Silvetri, cared for him during his last years. The two settled in Rome where, surprisingly, Cardano was favorably received by the College of Physicians. The Pope granted him a pension and Cardano continued writing his books. His last manuscript was De Propria Cita, the first medical autobiography to be written. Overall, Cardano published 131 works, burned 171 manuscripts he considered worthless, and kept 111 other books in manuscript. Cardano died at the age of seventy-four.

Judging Cardano's worth has been difficult for researchers. He was a superstitious man; but so were most men in his day. He was often a thoughtless man who made enemies easily. And yet he was a tremendously learned man in many areas of knowledge. And he was an excellent practitioner who worked with simple cures. The philosopher Leibnitz judged

5

him thus: "Cardano was a great man with all his faults; without them he would have been incomparable."[3]

ELLIOTSON

"A unanimous chorus of praise is not an assurance
of survival."[4]

Andre Gide

John Elliotson (1791-1868), appointed professor of the
practice of medicine in the University of London, was an
unrivaled clinical teacher and a prominent physician. He
distinguished himself by his many lectures and papers which
were regularly published in medical journals. He was the first
to practice auscultation and to use the stethoscope. He
founded the Phrenological Society and was elected president
of the Royal Medical and Chirurgical Society of London. He
also helped to establish the University College Hospital.
Because of his many accomplishments, Elliotson was considered one of London's most able physicians.

But at the same time, he was considered an eccentric, in
both his appearance and his interests. He wore a beard when
no one wore beards, and he refused to wear the customary
knee-breeches and silk stockings. He advocated unconventional theories and practices. Phrenology—the study of the
skull's conformation to determine character and mental capacity—was one of his many interests. He also experimented
with dosages of medicine, sometimes prescribing large doses
of drugs considered poisonous. And he protested the common
use of blood-letting for numerous ailments.

Elliotson was also concerned with unpopular social problems; the severity of the penal code; the lack of attention to the
mental health of criminals; the effects of overcrowding in
slums; the effects of poor sanitation; the establishment of an
educational system; etc. His attention to children was also
progressive, so much so that he is sometimes called the first
child therapist. He found that children received less attention
than criminals, mentally ill patients, or alcoholics. And the
attention they received, he said, was often cruel, resulting in

7

many childhood illnesses and disorders. Overwork and mis-handling by adults caused many of their behavioral and health problems. He suggested that children be sent to bed to rest for these conditions, instead of being whipped. Elliotson's interest in these uncommon ideas did not greatly interfere with his professional standing. But when he became involved with mesmerism, or hypnosis, this changed.

Elliotson first became interested in hypnosis in 1829. He deemed it a novelty that might prove useful and held public exhibitions in various homes to show the miraculous results of mesmerism on epileptic patients. Over the next nine or ten years he also used it in many experiments. With hypnosis he was successful in calming hysteria, then classified as a disease. (Later he contradicted his contemporaries' opinions that hysteria came from the womb, afflicting women only.) Another nervous disorder he successfully treated was St. Vitus' dance (Sydenham's chorea). He also cured some skin diseases and reported that he had helped several insane patients.

Elliotson's increasing absorption with hypnosis began to worry his fellow professors. They did not like the experiments he was conducting on the university hospital's patients. But when he published a paper on Numerous Cases of Surgical Operation without Pain in the Mesmeric State, they felt they could no longer overlook his activities. They banned the use of mesmerism in the university and its hospital, and then forced him to resign.

Soon after this, Elliotson and his followers started a quarterly called The Zoist which presented articles on many subjects, including hypnosis. The journal did have some influence on other doctors. Mesmeric hospitals and clinics were founded in Edinburgh, Dublin, Exeter, and with Elliotson's help, in London. Various doctors occasionally wrote about mesmerizing their surgical patients. But overall, physicians opposed Elliotson. He was called "a professional pariah" and a "madman," and his quarterly, an "infamous publication."[5] He lost most of his practice and many of his friends. Doctors who had consulted with him no longer sought his advise. Nonetheless he was able to continue his work, presenting exhibitions in various homes and treating patients in the Mesmeric Infirmary in London, although he always refused to call himself a mesmerist. He was simply a doctor, one of whose techniques was mesmerism, he said. Finally, his health failing him, and lacking finances to sufficiently support himself, he moved to the home of a former devoted student, Dr. E. S. Symes, where he died in 1868.

Although Elliotson was censured by the medical profession, there were others who realized his ability as a physician. Elliotson enjoyed the steady friendship of Charles Dickens, who was fascinated by the physician's innovations. An obscure writer, Overs, dedicated a collection of short stories to Elliotson for his long years of dedicated work, and Thackeray dedicated Pendennis (1850) to Elliotson's service. And so, Elliotson's devotion to medical care has not been totally forgotten.

HAMMOND

"In their blind anger men sacrifice their benefactors, and then deify them when convinced at last that no false prophet was there. It is the charlatan and the imposter that we fear; so we kill the man of good works, and later tell how he was no knave."[6]

James Mumford

For troops wounded in the early battles of the Civil War, medical attention was disastrous. At these battles, poor preparation, inadequate supplies, and bad teamwork overwhelmed many medical efforts. Regimental and regular army surgeons quarrelled about their authority and responsibilities, some caring only for the men under their command. Civilians hired as ambulance drivers led the retreats, usually leaving the wounded lying on the battlefield. Once it took a week to clear the field of the dead and wounded. Then there were serious problems in Washington where the Union Congress, penurious at best, refused to accept the realities of the war and the need for stockpiles of supplies. They were usually tardy in meeting the requisitions given them so that army doctors had to buy medicine from private sources. The surgeon-general was Thomas Lawson, a doddering old man, whose primary concern was to reduce his budget so that his annual outlay was kept close to $120,000. He died shortly after the start of the war but was replaced by another inept bureaucrat. After several bloody battles and grossly mismanaged medical care, the United States Sanitary Commission, a group of civilians concerned with the health of the troops, pressured Congress to reorganize the Medical Bureau.

Surgeon-General Finley was removed and Congress began its search for a new administrator. But the Medical Bureau was steeped in its own pettymindedness and conservatism. They wished to appoint the man next in line in seniority. The Commission, however, discovered a young man, William A.

11

Hammond, only thirty-four years old, who had compiled an outstanding record as a doctor. He had served eleven years as an army surgeon, and while on leave had observed hospitals and medical developments throughout Europe. He had published many papers, including an essay on the nutritive value of albumen, starch, and gum, for which he had received a prize from the American Medical Association. Because of his many accomplishments, he had won an enviable reputation as a forward-thinking physician and researcher. After several years as a professor at the University of Maryland, he reenlisted in the army with the Civil War's outbreak. The Commission saw in him the man they neeeded to reorganize the Medical Department. After much political wrangling and maneuvering, Hammond won his appointment as surgeon-general. He stepped up from captain to brigadier-general with this appointment, to the consternation of the many army surgeons between these ranks.

No sooner was Hammond in office than he began to clash with Secretary of War Stanton. The two men conflicted on their views of the medical organization. Stanton wanted a strongly centralized organization that would keep the power in his own hands. Hammond, on the other hand, wished to decentralize the department, giving qualified officers control over certain functions. Stanton delayed the appointment of Hammond's inspectors, directors, and assistants, and then nominated only half of Hammond's candidates, filling in the other positions with his own choices. He then warned Hammond to disassociate himself from the Sanitary Commission—a group of civilians concerned with the health of the troops—which he saw as a threat and an embarrassment to the Medical Bureau.

Hammond set to work. And the effects of his work were soon evident. In the 1862 fiscal year, the Medical Bureau had not even spent its budget of $2,445,000. The following year, Hammond's budget was $10,214,000 and its expenditure was $11,594,000. In a letter to the medical director of the Army of the Potomac, John Letterman, he explained his new policies. All red tape was to be disregarded. Only efficiency and results were important. If Letterman needed supplies, he was to order them—no limits. If he needed more doctors and nurses, he was to hire them—no need for authorization. Field surgeons would finally begin to get the personnel and supplies they so desperately needed.

The first major battle during Hammond's appointment was the Second Manassas of 1862. After the bloody battle, some wounded men were left on the battlefield for days. Hammond immediately demanded authorization to form an ambulance corps. But the Secretary of War and his supporters refused the project as too expensive. Medical Director Letterman did not listen to their veto, but under the authority of General McClellan organized an ambulance corps for his division. The system worked so well that it became the model for similar corps throughout the world. By the last year of the Civil War, it was also used in all divisions of the Union Army.

After six months' experience, Hammond formulated his list of desired reforms which he presented to the War Department. He again stressed the need for an ambulance corps and for special hospital staff, like cooks, nurses, and attendants. He requested more surgeons, and the authority to appoint medical cadets and employ civilian physicians. He also requested more inspectors and assistants.

Hammond's next recommendation was to establish a graduate school of medicine to continually update medical officers' knowledge of scientific advances. This would include a medical museum. He also proposed homes for disabled soldiers, an increase in rank and pay for surgeons, and a doubling of the funds for hospital rations.

The fate of these proposals was discouraging. Fifty surgeons and 250 assistant surgeons, whose commissions would lapse with the end of the war, was all the Congress saw necessary. Stanton objected to the idea of a graduate school with evening classes because students, he said, would cut their classes in favor of the theater. Such objections met each proposal.

Hammond then knew any reforms he wanted would have to be effected within the existing bureaucratic framework. He developed a system of patient case-cards that allowed better medical care. He reclassified diseases so that they incorporated medical advances. He developed the pavilion hospital building with ridge ventilation that kept the air fresh. He improved the Reserve Surgeons Corps, which answered the need for emergency personnel. He set up laboratories to manufacture medicines and test purchased drugs for purity. He also stockpiled supplies in numerous cities and bases.

Through all these changes, Hammond made his enemies. He had often effected the reforms bluntly and tactlessly, sometimes disregarding military policy. But one change outraged so many of the medical profession that his downfall was certain. He withdrew two drugs from the supply table, both of which were harmful but often used: calomel (mercurous chloride) and tartar emetic—both of which caused acute and chronic poisoning. The principle result of this announcement was an even greater dislike of Hammond.

Throughout his appointment Hammond had relied on the Sanitary Commission for supplies, for inspections, and for the gathering of statistics. This reliance only gained him the War Department's contempt. When the antagonism reached an intolerable point, Hammond was ordered away from Washington and Joseph Barnes named Acting Surgeon General. Hammond asked for a trial by court martial in which he was charged with unmilitary and ungentlemanly conduct. He was also charged with breaking military policy. All charges were without qualification. Hammond had not paid off debts from the Western medical corps, but prosecutors failed to mention that Stanton had denied Hammond the money. He was charged with making certain purchases against department policy, yet he had made them with Stanton's approval. He was charged with spending too much money on supplies, but prosecutors did not add that he did this after major battles for which there were inadequate supplies. The list of charges went on and on in this manner.

After a rather vicious battle, the court ruled in Stanton's favor. The court pronounced Hammond guilty of all charges. He was dismissed and barred from ever again holding a governmental position. Many protested the verdict, calling the trial vindictive and incomplete because of stolen or suppressed evidence. But their dissension did nothing to help his cause. Hammond left the army for New York City, where he assumed leadership in the teaching of neurology. While there he and his colleagues founded two post-graduate medical schools. In 1888 he returned to Washington where he founded a sanitarium for mental patients. He practiced there until his death in 1889.

Thirteen years after his court martial, Congress reviewed their action. They agreed that Hammond had been technically guilty of various charges. But they now understood his reasons for disregarding policy. They also saw that Hammond had instituted or called for all the improvements carried out during the war and, historians say, for the next three decades after the war. Hammond had accomplished all this in but fifteen months. Congress now exonerated him of all charges and restored his rank as retired brigadier-general and surgeon-general.

HUNT

"Expedient for us to enter hospitals as patients, but inexpedient for woman, however well qualified, to be there as a physician...The word inexpedient I had always abhorred—it is so shuffling, so shifting, so mean, so evasive...an apology for falsehood, a compromise of principle."[7]

Harriot Kezia Hunt

Harriot Hunt (1805-1875) opened a school for girls with her sister when her father died leaving the family in financial straits. In directing the school, Hunt saw the importance of proper sanitation and hygiene for the prevention of disease, and she began to study medical texts. Later she pursued her studies with an English doctor who had settled in Boston. With his tutelage, she read profoundly and diversely until she felt well enough prepared to open her own office. In 1835 she started her medical practice with her sister's help. Her practice without a degree was not unusual as many doctors did not have medical degrees. She became the first woman to practice medicine successfully in the United States, although not the first woman to receive her medical degree. The latter honor belongs to Elizabeth Blackwell.

Because she was not a licensed practitioner, she did not feel bound to the commonly accepted medical theories, although she saw the importance of a thorough medical education. Mental disease particularly interested her. She soon discovered that the cure of many physical ailments was "ministering to a mind diseased, or plucking from the memory a rooted sorrow."[8] She was also interested in helping women. She founded the Ladies' Physiological Society in Charlestown, where she lectured on disease prevention and proper hygiene for both the body and the mind. With her later interest in the women's rights movement, she began several lecture tours through Eastern states. Her topic was always "Woman as a

Physician to Her Sex." Her lectures benefited many women who rarely received frank information about their own physical health from male doctors.

Despite the success she later enjoyed in her practice, she had to overcome difficulties. She avoided housecalls at first because friends of her patients who saw that the doctor was a woman would greatly oppose her, neutralizing any benefit from her visit. She also had difficulties gathering necessary medical information. Although her studies had been as thorough as possible without a medical school education, Hunt still found cases she felt unprepared to accept. In 1847, at the age of forty-two and after twelve years of practice, she applied to Harvard Medical College for permission to attend the school's public lectures. She was refused because no female students were allowed. One month after Elizabeth Blackwell was accepted in Geneva Medical College, Hunt reapplied. Again she was rejected; this time the board found reconsideration "inexpedient." This refusal angered Hunt and caused her to align herself with the women's rights movement.

Three years later she again applied, pointing out that ideas were changing and that female physicians were more commonly accepted. This time the faculty voted to accept Hunt's application to attend lectures, although they would not grant her a degree. At this same meeting, they admitted three black men to the school. When the medical students heard of the four unusual admissions, they protested. They found the black men "repulsive," and they claimed that Hunt would undermine their dignity and self-respect. They refused to mix with this "unsexed" woman. The faculty reversed their decision.

Hunt never again applied to a medical school, although she did receive an honorary medical degree from The Women's Medical College of Philadelphia in 1853. She spent the next twenty years in active medical practice, always fighting for the acceptance of women not only in the medical profession, but also in other professions: "All women-workers have my

18

benediction," she said.[9] Despite a happy and fulfilled life, she always regretted and resented being deprived of a thorough medical education by the backward-thinking Harvard medical students.

HUNTER

"My fellow Creatures of the Hospital are a damn'd disagreeable set. The two Heads are as unfit for Employment, as the Devil was to reign in Heaven!"[10]

John Hunter

John Hunter (1728-1793), born in East Kilbride, Scotland, was always considered the schoolroom dullard. Teachers tried every method of reward and punishment to redeem him, but in exasperation they gave up. And so Hunter's mother took him out of school at the age of thirteen, ending the only formal education he would ever receive. He could barely write and showed little promise. He eventually traveled to London to help his brother William, a physician. William had lived and worked in London for some time and had rid himself of his Scottish accent and country bumpkin behavior and dress. And now here was John—unlettered, uncouth, pugnacious, and raw. But William needed an assistant, especially since the anatomy course he taught was about to begin, and it attracted as many as a hundred students. His prospectus advertised dissection as an important part of the course, so he had to procure scores of bodies. He delegated this responsibility to John—a wise choice for John talked the language of the body snatchers. He bought and accepted drinks, and even helped with the body-snatching. Soon he was given preferential treatment.

During this time, William allowed John to do some original research. John proved that the testicles, epididymis, and vas deferens formed a continuous passage. This was only the first of many experiments and discoveries. After several years' experience with William, John began to practice medicine, especially surgery. As he never learned Latin or passed the examination before the Corporation of Surgeons' Court of Examiners, John practiced without a license, which was fairly common in London at the time. John's academic shortcomings, however, always bothered him. He found it difficult to express himself clearly, either in speaking or writing. And because he had read very little about medicine, even in his own field, he sometimes was caught in weeks of needless effort solving a problem already solved. Nonetheless, in 1754 he was admitted as a surgeon's pupil to St. George's Hospital.

He was also very busy with a project that would fascinate him all his life: the anatomy of animals, especially rare breeds of animals. He began his lifetime collection of animals to anatomize. He owed enormous sums of money to petshop owners. He bribed zoo keepers to let him dissect some of the animals. He bought old, diseased animals from circus owners and rare show owners. He even convinced explorers to bring back animals and plants typical of distant lands. His collection included animals as common as the bee or the alley cat and as exotic as the poteroo or the tapua tafa.

In 1759 Hunter contracted pneumonia and decided to leave dissecting rooms and hospital wards for a while. He joined the army as a staff surgeon. During the various expeditions he was assigned to during the Seven Years' War, he was able to continue his anatomizing and embalming of strange marine life and reptiles. He also gained a reputation as a good surgeon. Not since Ambroise Paré had recommended new battlefield treatments had gunshot wound treatments been improved. Hunter now stated that not all bullets needed to be removed. He believed in the natural curative powers of the body upset by extensive surgery which could cause more hemorrhage, greater pain and shock, and increased risk of infection. He only extracted bullets when unavoidable. He also contributed an operation for aneurysm that saved thousands of lives and limbs. All this the other doctors watched with curiosity and often resentment. John, still as tactless and cocky as before, did not conceal his contempt for their traditional medical procedures. One time he so infuriated a fellow doctor that the man drew his sword.

Finally in 1763 Hunter returned to England laden with his notebooks, bones, and specimens. He was unable to work with his brother who had meanwhile hired another assistant. His only income was the meager army pension he received. He started to build up a rather small practice. But because he could not support himself, he allied himself with the Spences, a family of Scottish barbers and tooth-pullers. Dentistry in the 1700's was ranked lowest among the healing arts. Physicians would only refer a patient to a dentist when such care was unavoidable. The Spences wished to have a surgical consultant work with them. Hunter immediately consented as he saw an opportunity to learn more about a relatively unknown field. The result was the first scientific treatise on dentistry in English, and the most extensive written until his day. But Hunter received only ridicule for his work with those "quacks."

Hunter continued his own research as well. He was puzzled by veneral diseases which had been epidemic for centuries. Few understood the gradual progression of syphilis or the differences between syphilis and gonorrhea. Since many of Hunter's patients suffered from these diseases, he wished to learn more about them. He theorized that the two diseases were different manifestations of the same infection. Syphilis occurred when the skin of the penis was infected; gonorrhea, when the mucous membrane within the urethra was infected. To prove his contention, he punctured his foreskin and the head of his penis with a lancet he had just used to drain the sore of a patient who suffered from gonorrhea. If his theory was correct, he should contract syphilis. Soon the familiar lesion of syphilis appeared and his theory seemed to have been confirmed. Today, we understand that through a mischance, the patient he treated must have been suffering from both diseases. But Hunter was confident of his experiment and pushed it to its limits, allowing himself to suffer for three years while he kept careful notes of the disease's progress. Finally he applied the optimum dosage of mercury and the lesions disappeared. Unknown to him, the syphilis remained, proceeding to ruin his health. Soon thereafter Hunter married. The early deaths and poor health of all his children have led researchers to question whether he did not transmit the disease to his wife and children.

The fallacy of his research with venereal disease slowed the investigation of venereal diseases for fifty years, until 1838 when a French dermatologist, Philippe Ricord, was finally able to prove that gonorrhea and syphilis were two separate diseases. But Hunter's work was not without value. His Treatise on Venereal Disease allowed the subject to be discussed more openly, less superstitiously and disparagingly. Although his conclusions were incorrect, his descriptions of the two diseases were accurate. The hard or Hunterian chancre was the departure point for all future investigators.

During his experiment, Hunter had begun to lecture at St. George's Hospital where he was at long last a member of the surgical staff. But he was still terrified of audiences and had to drink a laudanum-port wine mixture before his lectures. His rather colloquial speech—"The ball having gone into the man's belly and hit his guts such a damn's thump, they mor-r-r-tified"[11]—and his lack of ease resulted in very small audiences, but gradually a band of young men rallied around him who embraced his revolutionary teachings. Hunter contended that surgery must be performed only when absolutely necessary, and then only after the whole patient had been considered—"his life history, habits, constitutional idiosyncrasies, and previous ailments; the structure and function of his organs in health; the systemic changes at the onset and during the course of the disease, and those likely to accompany the postoperative and convalescent states; the interactions of his mind, emotions, and body."[12] Hunter was especially interested in the last consideration because he was aware of the psychological factors in disease and the powers of the mind. He also claimed that surgeons were too concerned with the facts rather than with the unknown principles underlying disease. Surgeons, he said, must be more concerned with causes.

These heretical ideas alienated the majority of Hunter's colleagues. They had no more patience for these and other strange ideas which included the first correct explanation of inflammation, the discovery of antisepsis a century before Lister, and his heretical concept of the world's age based on geological evidence rather than religious doctrine. They had long derided his careful collection of specimens of every kind of animal. On his property, which he called Earls Court, he had created a museum with thousands of plant and animal preparations. He called this museum his unwritten book to the world. But few of his contemporaries saw any reason for his collection and failed to see in his work a major contribution to the science of comparative anatomy. He was the joke of London and was even lampooned by William Blake. But Hunter's manner did not help matters. His colleagues always remembered his comment that he was a pygmy in knowledge, and yet a giant compared to them.

Hunter soon felt the weight of his colleagues' enmity. One group even hired a man named Jesse Foot to write a defamatory biography about Hunter. Foot, egged on by a personal grudge against him, scavenged for all the sordid details he could find in order to discredit Hunter. Much of this he received from other surgeons at St. George's Hospital. This book appeared under the innocent title of The Life of John Hunter.

With the mounting tension Hunter's health deteriorated. He suffered a severe attack of angina pectoris from which he never fully recovered. Any exertion could induce spasms. And as he grew older he was prone to violent rages that only further provoked his attacks—both possibly the result of advanced syphilis. The physicians now took advantage of his weakness, spreading scandalous rumors about his practice, attempting to refute all his ideas and innovations. One doctor even claimed that he watched one of Hunter's patients die after an operation for aneurysm. But he failed to mention that the patient died over a year later from unrelated causes. Physicians at St. George's also closed ranks against Hunter because he charged them with irresponsibility to students and patients.

In 1790 Hunter was temporarily drawn into another difficult situation. He was appointed surgeon-general. He decided to reform and reorganize the army medical corps. He would not allow the previous patronage of dispensing commissions to favorites of the members of Parliament. Commissions now had to be earned after a term of service in the lower ranks. With this new resolution, he created a whole new set of enemies. But during the war he was able to direct the medical corps successfully as well as continue his private practice, his lectures, and his research.

He could not, however, maintain this pace for long. The physicians at St. George's ruled that students could be accepted only if they brought a certificate of previous related education. This new ruling was sure to exclude many Scots who came to study under Hunter. In October, 1793, two young Scots without certificates tried to enter the hospital. Hunter tried to intercede for them at a board meeting. All present realized the pain he suffered and the precariousness of his health, but this did not stop them from rudely interrupting his speech. Hunter struggled to control his temper and staggered into an adjoining room where he collapsed. He died later that day.

Hunter was buried without ceremony or official honors. His colleagues did not pass a vote of condolence. The minutes of the next board meeting recorded that "one of the surgeons" had died. The press almost forgot to mention him. And when his wife asked that he be buried at Westminster Abbey, she won no support. Sixty-six years later an army surgeon who had long respected Hunter found the doctor's coffin and transferred it to Westminster Abbey where it was reinterred, next to Ben Jonson's burial place, with proper ceremony.

Although Hunter made no single great discovery, his vast research in anatomy and physiology raised surgery to the level of a distinct branch of science. And many have called him the founder of surgical pathology. But for his years of service and contribution, he received no recognition. Fortunately today we understand his place in medical history.

LIND

"The thoroughness of the reformer's victory...is that which most makes silence of the reformer's fame."[13]

Sir John Simon

The change from oars to sails as the primary means of propelling ships profoundly affected health and sanitation at sea. This was even more true when the mast and sail were fully developed, because they allowed long oceanic voyages. Oar-propelled vessels hugged the shorelines and were always able to obtain fresh provisions, and seafaring diseases, such as scurvy, seldom occurred. But sailing vessels could venture far from land and thus depended on salted and preserved foods. And so, seafaring diseases became rampant. These larger ships also needed a larger crew. So the number of decks and compartments was increased, causing inadequate ventilation. Respiratory and contagious diseases resulted, particularly in voyages to the tropics, where so many new diseases were encountered.

Of all the diseases, however, scurvy took one of the heaviest tolls. This was directly related to the men's diet. The standard ration for the British Royal Navy in the 1700's consisted of biscuits, salted meat, dried fish, cheese, peas, butter, and beer. This provided adequate calories but few vitamins, especially vitamin C.

Physicians as early as 1590 recognized the value of citrus fruits in preventing and treating scurvy. One of these was John Woodall, born in 1570. Woodall, a prominent physician, was appointed to the position of surgeon-general of the East India Company. In 1617, he published The Surgeon's Mate, a manual for all the surgeons in the Company. In it he advised that lemon juice be carried on all voyages to treat scurvy. And when landing in the Indies, the ships' surgeons were to persuade their pursers to buy oranges, limes, lemons, or tamarinds for the crews. Woodall's advise was followed by the East India Company with great success, but before the end of the century, his lessons were forgotten. In fact, during the two centuries from 1600 to 1800, when a prevention for scurvy was known, one million sailors died from scurvy; this is but a conservative estimate, which, when added to the number of those who recovered from inadequate vitamin C, would present an even more dreadful picture of the problem.

This needless loss of men affected many expeditions and military battles to the point of threatening national security. Four to five thousand deaths a year from scurvy in the navy influenced all major naval battles between 1600 and 1800. Herbert Spencer noted that "the mortality from scurvy during this long period had exceeded the mortality by battles, wrecks, and all casualties of sea-life put together!"[14]

In addition to Woodall, another significant spokesman for the use of citrus fruits and juices in the navy was James Lind (1716-1794). Up to his time more than eighty books and papers on scurvy had been published. Many of these recommended the use of citrus fruits. It seems that many seafarers who had had much to do with scurvy were convinced that the illness was due to the lack of fresh foods. And yet, all these spokesmen were largely ignored. And Lind, too, went unheeded for some time.

Lind gained his first medical experience as an apprentice to a prominent physician. When he turned twenty-three, he joined the Naval Medical Service, spending the next ten years at sea, much of it in the tropics. He was appalled by the conditions under which the men lived at sea—airless cabins, overcrowding, darkness and dampness, diets of rancid meat and moldy biscuits, and countless diseases, the most frequent of which was scurvy.

In May of 1747 while on the seventy-four gun ship Salisbury, Lind decided to experiment with various scurvy treatments. He chose twelve patients in similar condition. He divided these into pairs. He then gave each pair different treatments: a quart of cider each day; elixir vitriol; vinegar; sea water; an electary of garlic, horse radish, gum myrrh, etc.; citrus fruits. The results were interesting. The men given the citrus fruits convalesced rapidly, one fit for duty after only six days. The next most effective cure was the cider. The remaining treatments did not improve the patients' health. This experiment—called the Salisbury experiment—demonstrated the preeminence of citrus fruits as a cure for scurvy.

In 1748, Lind left the Navy to take his degree at the University of Edinburgh. He then set up his practice in the city, meanwhile working on his book, A Treatise on the Scurvy, which was published in 1753 and later went through three editions. The work, containing a description of the Salisbury experiment and dedicated to one of the commissioners of the Admiralty, went unnoticed. Nevertheless, Lind was much respected by his peers who elected him Fellow and Treasurer of the Royal College of Physicians in Edinburgh. He was then appointed physician to the King's Royal Hospital at Haslar where he remained for twenty-five years.

During this time he treated thousands of scurvy victims. He was able to continue his citrus fruit research which he incorporated into the third edition of his treatise. He also worked to right many of the misconceptions passed on by a Dutch physician, Severius Eugalenus, whose work on scurvy, first published in 1588, was still popular during Lind's lifetime. Eugalenus confused the symptoms of scurvy with those of other diseases. He also taught a procedure of diagnosis— taking the patient's pulse—which led him to conclude that most everyone suffered from scurvy. This he attributed to God's anger at man's sinfulness. Lind's findings, based on experiment and observation, directly attacked Eugalenus' theories which were so widely accepted. Unfortunately, Lind went unheard.

Lind did not restrict himself to the study of scurvy, however. He pioneered other innovations as well. He wrote a book about preserving the health of sailors. In it he included suggestions for improving the comfort and morale of the crew. He recommended the use of receiving ships to assure the health of the sailors. Here they would be examined, kept for a period of observation and seasoning, and issued standard uniforms. He recommended and explained the distillation of sea water to insure fresh, pure water rather than the putrid water brought from shore in casks which caused epidemics of typhoid, cholera, and dysentery. And since resuscitation of the apparently drowned sailor was essential to naval surgeons, he described several methods of resuscitation. Then, he was the first to develop and use a concentrated emergency ration for boats or rafts. In another treatise on tropical diseases (1768)—the first book published on this topic since 1598— Lind discussed many of the problems Europeans encounter with a hot, humid climate. He recommended various actions to avoid mosquito bites and prevent malaria. He also made accurate observations on tetanus, polyneuritis, and other diseases.

All of these developments secured Linds' position as a well respected physician. He occupied the remainder of his life with his research and clinical work. Lind resigned from Haslar in 1783. He continued his studies in naval and tropical medicine until his death in 1794.

Forty years after Lind's death, his prevention for scurvy was finally put into practice. All ships were required to carry lemon juice or limes on board (hence the term "limey" for the British sailor). The effects of his methods were widespread. For example, in the battle of Quiberon Bay, special ships carried fresh provisions to Sir Edward Hawke's fleet during their blockade. Out of 14,000 men, not even twenty were on the sick list on the day of the battle despite months of arduous service. Not only were the effects seen in military actions, but also in merchant commerce and even in Arctic explorations. Scurvy was all but wiped out, due to the efforts of many men, but especially Lind, a pioneer in naval medicine and hygiene who has been forgotten because the effect of his work was so

32

complete. For decades much of his work was ignored, to the detriment of thousands of seamen. But fortunately, the worth of his methods was discovered and countless more lives saved.

MALPIGHI

"I live, if you can call such inactivity living...I
have no other aim but that of distracting my
thought away from my loss."[15]

Marcello Malpighi

Born near Bologna, Italy, Marcello Malpighi (1628-
1694) traveled to the nearby University of Bologna to work on
his doctor of medicine degree. There he was considered the
school's most brilliant student. But in his doctor's thesis, he
took a position his professors could not accept. He con-
demned some of the teachings of the ancient physicians
Galen, Avicenna, and Rhases. His professors rejected his
thesis. Not until he removed all condemnatory remarks was
his paper finally accepted and his degree granted. But some
of the professors protested this. They did not like the idea of
graduating from their university a student who doubted and
suspected the ancients' long-upheld teachings. They succeeded in having Malpighi's diploma recalled, and only after
a lengthy battle in which Malpighi was supported by a powerful professor was his diploma returned.

Although Malpighi could now start a practice, he decided
against this for he disliked dealing with patients. Instead, he
soon became quite well-known for his research and was even
appointed lecturer at the university. But his detractors kept up
their attacks: his lectures were stopped; derogatory rumors
and statements dogged him.

Finally Malpighi decided that he could no longer endure
these attacks and accepted a position at the University of Pisa,
a newer school which certainly promised more open-minded-
ness. But there the oppressive humidity caused him grave
health problems, and with the counsel of Massari, a supportive
former professor, he returned to Bologna. But the situation
had not changed. Intrigues were ever-constant. Upon the advice of another friend, he traveled to Messina, Sicily. Profes-

sors and physicians in Messina, however, were even more backward in their thinking.

In order to communicate his ideas without such fear of censure, Malpighi was forced to start sharing his ideas with doctors in universities throughout Europe. His letters in Latin traveled to distant countries where his reputation was slowly being formed. These letters told of his research with a microscope he himself had constructed. Malpighi had over the years recorded his careful and accurate observations. He had described and sketched the network of tiny blood vessels in a frog's mesentery. He had even seen the blood corpuscles moving through these vessels. He had shown how the blood flowed through the frog's body. He had also demonstrated that the trachea divided into bronchi which underwent a series of division ending in tiny hollow cells surrounded by a network of blood vessels. He had seen that the inspired air and the blood were separated by fine membranes. Malpighi had also added to the knowledge of other organs, especially of the spleen and liver. He had described red blood cells and pioneered the field of microscopic embryology. News of these discoveries and observations traveled far.

But former students and professors from Bologna still would not accept him. One published a book entitled Triumph of the Galenians, which re-emphasized the importance of Galen's teachings and the study of drugs. Bending over a microscope was considered merely an idle pastime. With this, Malpighi's patience gave out. He collected a list of Galen's errors, and point by point showed how his work had rectified them. He returned to Bologna to publish this booklet and decided to remain in the city he considered home. But old hostilities took up once again. His lectures were rudely interrupted, his teachings berated. Finally Malpighi retired to a villa close to Bologna where he could carry on his work without further nuisance. He was greatly respected throughout Europe, but, spurned in his own city.

Although many Bologna professors denounced him, one

in particular was very bitter. Girolamo Sbaragli was a Galenist physician and an enemy of the Malpighi family because of an ancient feud that had originated in a property dispute; each generation had carried on this vendetta. Marcello Malpighi and Girolamo Sbargli now took up the cudgels. The clash between ideology as well as between families made this dispute especially fierce.

Sbarabli published a booklet, <u>Study of Contemporary Physicians</u>, which claimed that microscopic research did nothing to further man's fight against disease, that such work was only the hairsplitting work of a pedant. Malpighi was forced to defend his life's work. In a long letter he exposed many errors in his opponent's thoughts and methods and clearly won this round. Sbarabli was infuriated by his loss.

He remembered the death of a relative by the hand of Malpighi's younger brother. And so in 1689, on a still June night, he and some masked followers burst in to Malpighi's study where the older doctor was once again peering through his microscope. Malpighi was mocked as the men pranced around him, singing derisive songs; furniture was overturned; microscopes and slides were destroyed; and Malpighi and his wife were injured. And then the men left. Shortly thereafter, the villa caught fire. All of Malpighi's books, his plant and insect collections, and all his data were burned.

This experience so wearied him of life that he withdrew for four years and wrote nothing. His friends saw that he was allowing himself to die. They sent word to the newly elected Pope, a friend of Malpighi's. The Pope invited the doctor to Rome to be his personal physician. After several entreaties Malpighi finally went. There he lived for the next three years. Before his death he entrusted the remainder of his papers to the Royal Society and left word that he wished to be dissected after his death so that he might still be of use to science.

After Malpighi's death, his students waited thirty hours to be sure he was dead. They found that blood vessels in his brain had broken. Blood vessels had brought Malpighi to fame and also to his deathbed.

MORGAN

"The wounds that are given by the envenomed
tongue of calumny are deeper and more fatal than
the sword. They destroy what is dearer than life
itself, reputation and peace of mind."[16]

John Morgan

John Morgan, born in 1735 into a wealthy Quaker family,
grew up in one of the colonies' leading cities, Philadelphia. A
year before graduation from Benjamin Franklin's College of
Philadelphia, Morgan apprenticed himself to a doctor—the
only way of studying medicine in the colonies. He later
became an apothecary for the first public hospital in America,
which was founded by Franklin and Dr. Thomas Bond. In
1758 he resigned from this position and accepted the commission of lieutenant in a regiment comprised of Franklin's pioneer fighting group, the Associators. Although he had been
commissioned as a combat officer, he soon found himself
taking on the duties of regiment surgeon. After three years of
fighting in the French-Indian Wars, he traveled to Europe to
study medicine. Because of Franklin's influence, Morgan
was able to study with London's leading anatomists. He then
traveled to Edinburgh to attend the preeminent medical school
there. Morgan proved himself a brilliant student. His graduation thesis on the nature of pus, a subject much debated,
recognized that pus came from the blood, not from solid
tissue, as many thought. One hundred years later Cohnhiem
proved this contention.

Morgan traveled on to continental Europe. In Paris, the
Royal Academy of Surgery, impressed by his anatomical and
histological knowledge, elected him to their fellowship. In
Rome his visit with a world-renowned anatomist who founded
pathology, Margagni, earned him membership in the Society
of Belles Lettres. After other travels throughout Europe visiting with dignitaries, such as the Pope, the King of Sardinia,

39

and Voltaire, he returned to Great Britain where he was elected Fellow of the Royal Society of London, member of the College of Physicians of Edinburgh, and Licentiate of the College of Physicians of London. All these honors were bestowed on him before he was twenty-eight years old.

During these European tours Morgan had plenty of time to consider colonial America's medical training. He clearly saw its many shortcomings. He decided to propose a new medical education for America; he saw that a "university establishment would be necessary, capable of teaching all branches of medical science, of making rigid requirements for entrance and graduation, and of giving valuable degrees."[17] He wrote down his plan, submitting it to Thomas Penn, the Proprietor of Pennsylvania, asking Penn to inform the College of Philadelphia's trustees of his proposal and to recommend him as founder of this medical school.

In 1765 Morgan returned to America full of his new, exciting ideas. He had received the highest medical honors possible, and now he was to present his plan for a medical school to the trustees. First, he insisted on pre-medical studies. Until this time any unlearned man could call himself a doctor if he aided a physician for a short time. But Morgan called for much more: Knowledge of languages, mathematics, biology, chemistry, and theory and practice of medicine. Second, he called for one year of practice at the Pennsylvania Hospital, after which candidates would receive the degree of Bachelor of Medicine. To become Doctors of Medicine, they would have to practice medicine for three years and then return to write theses. Third, Morgan advocated specialization in medicine. A physician should not be expected to be doctor, apothecary, surgeon, and dentist, he said. He especially opposed physicians who made their living by dispensing drugs. Leave that to the apothecaries, he said, and practice medicine. To offset this loss in income and the greater investment in education, Morgan proposed that doctors should be paid more than was customary. All of these

40

ideas Morgan presented to the trustees who respected his thinking, but considered it in some ways too advanced.

A childhood friend of Morgan's, William Shippen, openly opposed Morgan. Shippen had been considered the outstanding young doctor of Philadelphia before Morgan's arrival. He too had been a brilliant medical student and after returning to his home in Philadelphia had attempted to improve medical training. But his plans had not been heeded, and so he had founded a private school of anatomy and obstetrics which the College had endorsed but not financially supported. He thus was angered by the attention Morgan received, especially when he found that John Morgan, at the age of twenty-nine, was appointed the head of the first medical school in America. The enmity and jealousy Shippen felt were to follow the two men from that time on.

Both Shippen and Morgan were appointed professors for the new medical school's first session. But Shippen claimed that, because he had been first to call for educational reform, he should direct the school. Morgan, however, retained his position. Soon the two men had their own factions of supporters. One historian sees the controversy as a bid for medical control in Philadelphia. The Shippens were an old line family, politically powerful; the Morgans an "upstart" family, financially comfortable. Morgan's "elevation to the foremost position in Philadelphia medicine was as a red cape to a bull in the eyes of the old line families."[18]

In 1775, ten years later, American independence was declared, and the Revolution began. Morgan was most influential in the colonies by now and particularly in the College of Physicians. He had married into an old line family and his father-in-law was politically powerful. Shippen's family was also politically powerful. But when Washington began his search for a doctor to command the army's medical services, he had no question as to whom to choose. Morgan was appointed director-general of military medicine—much to Shippen's anger—both because of his medical career and

41

because of his early military experience.

As Morgan reviewed the medical conditions of the Army, he saw that they were horrible. Regimental surgeons were incompetent, untrained men who received their commissions because of political influence. These same surgeons openly defied Morgan's predecessor's system which called for the slightly ill to be treated at the poorly equipped regimental hospitals and the seriously ill to be sent to the more adequate general hospitals. These surgeons did as they wished, flouting regulations, dissipating hard-to-find drugs and surgical instruments, and refusing to be held accountable for their requisitions; record-keeping was impossible. Some surgeons were even selling scarce medicines to the British. Morgan saw that these problems resulted from the lack of discipline in the medical branch of the Army.

And so he ruthlessly set to work, demanding discipline and accountability and developing a qualifying examination for all regimental surgeons, some of whom resigned upon hearing this. He also announced that he intended to use his supply of drugs wisely and frugally and re-emphasized the need for the seriously ill to be sent to the larger hospitals. Needless to say, he was poorly received. As the war continued, conditions grew worse: epidemics raged, drugs were scarce, hospitals became places to die. But Morgan found no support for his improvements. He constantly communicated with Congressman Samuel Adams' medical committee, but its members were too busy to help him or to answer his pleas for medicine, instruments, and good surgeons. So Morgan began his frequent rides covering hundreds of miles in search of medicine and sheets for bandages. Soon he was informed that workmen who had manufactured instruments were assigned to arms manufacturing. The Congress passed a bill forcing Morgan to dispense all of his own supplies that he had collected and thriftily doled out. But a second clause in the bill seemed a beginning; it made surgeons accountable to Morgan. This so angered the surgeons that they began to

42

spread rumors of incompetency and atrocity about Morgan. They blamed Morgan for all the deaths in the hospitals. Morgan responded with contempt for these men, which only increased insubordination and their dislike for him. Morgan saw that their lack of discipline was killing the troops: they refused to dig privies, so troops were dying of dysentery. But Congress gave him no means to take effective action.

Meanwhile, Morgan was unaware that his enemies were beginning to rally against him. Shippen was particularly active in this, so much so that he was elected surgeon to a small camp in New Jersey under Morgan's orders. He immediately wrote to Morgan asking his advice on military medicine—at the same time writing a series of letters to Congress aggrandizing his own achievements. He boasted that all his wounded were recovering, that only 10 to 12 out of 20,000 to 30,000 had died—all untrue. But Congress believed his reports and thought him more capable than his superior. So they gave him complete command over all the hospitals on the New Jersey side of the Hudson.

Morgan, arriving in New Jersey without knowledge of this, immediately started setting up a hospital. Three hundred sick and wounded were brought to him. He had no staff, no bread, no flour, no provisions, etc. He sent off dispatch-riders and cared for the sick alone for one week. Finally doctors arrived and Morgan that day galloped to Fort Lee for supplies. Shippen met him there informing him that he, Shippen, was now in command in New Jersey. Morgan—angry, hysterical, exhausted—could not believe that this had happened.

But Shippen was not yet content. He wrote to Congress further denigrating Morgan. Soon many started to blame Morgan for the rampant disease and lack of supplies. He became the scapegoat for all their losses. The conflict came to a head when Dr. Samuel Springer, in charge of medical affairs in northern New York, openly defied Morgan, who courtmartialed him and dismissed him. But Springer had political backing. Together he, Shippen, and their supporters were politically formidable. Congress could not overlook their complaints. Congress heard Morgan charged with all the medical disasters and misdeeds. Soon some congressmen were even saying that Morgan's presence was a threat to Army enlistment. Morgan heard all of this. He went to Philadelphia, where Samuel Adams advised him to resign because he had been charged with gross negligence and incompetence. Morgan refused. He demanded a chance to answer these charges but was allowed none. Shortly after attempting to help Washington, who had fought the Battle of Trenton without the hospital department—Shippen's responsibility—he received a curt discharge from the Army. And Shippen jubilantly accepted his new appointment as director-general to the Army medical services.

A shattered Morgan returned to Philadelphia. Over the next months, he tried to persuade Congress to hear his defense, but it would not listen. He finally published his Vindication in which he included documents, statements, and correspondence in his defense. He also called for an investigation. He rode throughout the countryside where he had served, gathering evidence in his own defense. He then appeared before the investigating committee, which completely vindicated him.

A loyal friend and former student of his, Benjamin Rush, helped him to courtmartial Shippen, who had allowed the medical department to deteriorate because of neglect. But despite convincing evidence of Shippen's dishonesty and disinterest in the Army's medical care, Shippen was acquitted. Once again Morgan and Rush prosecuted Shippen. This time the evidence must have been overwhelming for court members who sympathized with Morgan were replaced with Shippen's supporters. Other members were threatened. Shippen was again acquitted but this time only by a majority of one vote. Shippen then resigned from his post as director-general supposedly at Washington's request. His wrongdoing— neglect of duty, misappropriation of funds, sale of supplies to enemies—must have been quite well-known.

Morgan had hoped that these last three years of vindication and courtmartials would revive his spirits, but he found his honor and self-esteem destroyed. He soon lived in brooding solitude. His home had been destroyed in the Revolution. His wife had died. He had severed his relationship with the medical school. In 1789, Benjamin Rush was called to Morgan's home and found him dead.

Shippen never regained the position in Philadelphia medicine he had once had. In fact, it was Rush who became Philadelphia's leading physician. However, Shippen had the power to destroy Morgan's two major contributions: his progress in military medicine and his dream for medical education. Shippen was disturbed by the competition of newly founded medical schools that demanded more of their students. He abolished the degree of Bachelor of Medicine and the pre-medical requirements, bestowing the doctor's degree on unfit, ill-educated men. Not until Johns Hopkins University was founded were pre-medical requirements reintroduced.

Unfortunately, Morgan lived long enough to see his lifetime work devastated.

PARÉ

"The envious praise that which they can surpass;
that which surpasses them they censure."[19]

Caleb C. Colton

In the sixteenth century, military surgery was quite bar-
baric. The common method of treating gunshot wounds was
to apply boiling elder oil to the wound. Other procedures were
equally harsh. After amputation, arteries were cauterized with
red-hot irons. No surgeon questioned these long-accepted
procedures until Ambroise Paré (c.1510-1590).

Paré started his studies in a barber shop (barber-surgeons
were commonly accepted) and worked later as a companion-
surgeon in Hotel Dieu in Paris. He gained most of his vast experience, however, as a military surgeon in the Italian campaigns, 1536-1545. It was there that he began to question the
rule of established treatments. After one lengthy battle, Paré
ran out of the boiling oil he used for gunshot wounds. To
replace it, he concocted a salve of egg yolks, attar of roses, and
turpentine which he spread over the wounds—a relief to the
men expecting the torture of the boiling oil. The next morning
he saw that those treated with the salve felt little pain, suffered
no inflammation, and had slept peacefully. Those treated with
the oil were in great pain, suffered inflammation, and were
feverish. He quickly discarded the oil treatment. He also
refused to cauterize arteries when he found a more effective
and humanitarian method for stopping the bleeding. He
revived the use of ligature after reading about the process in
Galen's writings.

In 1575 Paré published these and other innovative surgical techniques, writing in French since he knew no Latin. The
powerful Faculté de Medecine immediately retaliated. They
ridiculed this upstart who did not know the learned man's
language and who was gaining respect because of his unorthodox procedures. They then tried to ban the publication of his

47

book because of an old decree allowing no medical book to appear in print without the Faculté's approval. Many other charges were brought against Paré as well, including plagiarism and corruption of morals. By the time the edict was reaffirmed, however, Paré's book had already been published and was selling particularly well because of his trial's publicity. Paré went on to topple other unfounded medical practices, publishing a discourse which stated that mummies and unicorns were worthless remedies although much prescribed by Parisian professors.

Paré's fame as a surgeon increased as he continued to make contributions through his observations. With his fame came increasing jealousy of his colleagues, who even attempted to poison him. One particularly scornful doctor, Etienne Gourmelen, published a book on surgery which attacked Paré's methods, especially ligature which he said opposed all the advice of the ancients. Paré countered with another edition of his work which explained that Hippocrates, Galen, Avicenna, and numerous others had explained and advised ligature. He also published a book defending his techniques and then describing his surgical experience in various military campaigns. He stressed the fact that he had obtained his knowledge in actual experience on the battlefield, whereas Gourmelen relied on his textbook for knowledge. Paré addressed Gourmelen directly: "Dare you teach me surgery... You who have never come out of your study. Surgery is learned by the eye and hand. You, mon petit maitre, know nothing else but how to chatter in a chair."[20]

Paré was eventually given the rank and the long robe of the master surgeon after serving as Henri II's chief surgeon. He gained considerable fame and was a surgeon much trusted despite the continued animosity of the Faculté de Medecine who, for years after, refused to accept his methods.

PINEL

"Science does not progress by traditional beliefs, but rather by radical new ideas of single, imaginative minds."[21]

Philip S. Callahan

Hippocrates helped to give medicine a scientific basis by replacing magic with careful observation. One particular medical field he advanced was that of mental health. He was the first to correctly describe neurosis with phobias, delirium accompanying various diseases, acute mental confusion following a severe hemorrhage, and other mental conditions. All of these, Hippocrates said, have a natural cause, whether physical or psychological. And nature can heal many of these illnesses if not interfered with. His theories, however, were lost to the mystics and magicians popular with the Greeks and Romans. Hippocrates' rational approach to mental illness had no place in their world.

The rise of Christianity in the superstitious Middle Ages further harmed this little understood medical field. The superstitious lore claimed that the moon drove people mad, hence the words lunacy and lunatic. Medieval Christianity did not help matters with its intolerant attitude toward those who were different. This intolerance led to a chaotic striving to destroy heresies and heretics, as in the mass witch hunts which persisted for three hundred years. Many a lunatic was burned at the stake in the name of God.

Fortunately the Age of Reason followed and psychiatry, devoted to the study of the mind, began to divest itself of supernaturalism. During the 1600's and 1700's, French monks founded more than a dozen asylums; secular groups also founded asylums. Even Paris's Hotel-Dieu had a special ward for the mentally ill. Its treatment program, lasting six weeks, consisted of baths, showers, bloodletting, blistering, and purgatives. If the patient did not progress with this

49

treatment he was transferred to either Bicetre, a men's asylum, or Salpetriere, a women's asylum. These institutions held all types: the poor, blind, epileptic, senile, criminal, and mentally ill. The wealthy never sent their own to these institutions, but rather to petites maisons or small hospitals of only twenty to thirty patients. The two large Parisian asylums, wretched one-way hospitals, were avoided by all who had the money to do so. But it was to Bicetre and Salpetriere that Philippe Pinel (1745-1826) devoted much of his life.

Pinel, born in south-central France, at first decided to become a priest, taking minor orders in a cathedral group. But after studying several years at the University of Toulouse and receiving his degree with honors, he decided to study medicine. He traveled to Montpellier, a medical school with an excellent reputation. While at Montpellier, Pinel became friends with Jean A. Chaptal, an intelligent but unhappy young man. Chaptal was confused about his life's direction and could not concentrate on any of his heavy curriculum. Pinel decided to help his friend by reading daily with him from Montaigne, Plutarch, and Hippocrates. Slowly Chaptal began to decide upon his goals, his aimless drifting stopped when he began to work toward these goals. Chaptal eventually succeeded in both science and politics. Pinel's psychological therapy probably started with this friendship.

While continuing further studies in Paris, Pinel began to write numerous articles on mental illness. And he looked into the newest theories and practices that might benefit the mentally ill. Mesmerism interested him, although he researched it carefully because of his own skepticism. Meanwhile he had begun to practice medicine; he still had to pass his oral licensing examination. Pinel was extremely shy, and had great difficulty speaking in public. He took the examination several times before he learned how to deal with this handicap.

But he forgot his own problems when a close friend became seriously mentally ill and, after running into the woods one day, was attacked and devoured by wolves. Pinel

50

now saw a clear direction for his life: he would devote his life to careful observation and treatment of mental illness. As he published more and more articles concerning his theories and treatments, he began to attract notice. Although he was not in sympathy with the revolutionary government, he was appointed head of Bicetre in 1793.

The conditions he found there were deplorable. The hospital itself was a huge fortress with barred windows and massive bolted doors. The courtyard was surrounded by insurmountable walls. Gutters in the stone floors of the cells carried off refuse which filled the air with an unbearable stench. Some patients were confined to cages, others to cells with a pen-like bed covered with straw, a restraining chair, and a toilet that could be emptied from the outside.

Naked or poorly dressed men were in chains attached to the floors and ceilings, and they lay on straw which was rarely changed. A tiny hole guarded by an iron grill was their sole link to the outside. Through this hole came their food and water and their physicians' diagnoses and recommendations for treatment. Because of the filth, skin infections covered their bodies. The attendants who cared for the inmates were unsympathetic men known for their uncommon strength, as all feared the supposed strength of madmen. Each attendant was assigned thirty to fifty patients and could use whatever methods he chose to protect himself.

These horrid conditions only worsened the patients' condition and they screamed for help, argued with everyone, and tried to destroy whatever they could within reach. For years the annual death rate hovered between one third and one half of the inmate population. Fifty-seven out of 110 died in 1784, and 95 out of 151 in 1788. But perhaps worst of all, Bicetre, a hell to those inside, was a tourist attraction to those outside who could amuse themselves by visiting the hospital. The attendants, for a small fee, would exhibit their patients.

To this place Pinel came and immediately brought change. First, he put an end to the starvation diet and to the tourist

51

visits. He did not believe, as most others did, that the mentally ill were evil creatures who merited abuse or punishment and needed to be guarded like wild beasts. He believed that mental illness is curable, and so proposed a radical change. He decided to remove the chains from some of the patients and institute an administration based on kindness and psychological therapy. This has been called le geste de Pinel or Pinel's grand geste. With it he advanced and humanized psychiatric treatment.

Before Pinel could institute this reform he needed the permission of the second revolutionary government, which distrusted him for his moderate political views. George Couthon was the leader of the Commune and suspected Pinel from the start, claiming that the doctor was hiding enemies of the state at Bicetre. Couthon even attempted to question the inmates and finally decided that Pinel was sincere but mad himself to unchain those "animals." But he gave Pinel permission.

The doctor carefully chose his first group of patients to free. The patients were ecstatic. One man imprisoned for forty years was taken outside and could not believe the sight of the sun. Before, all were afraid to approach him because he had killed an attendant who had cruelly provoked him. This man was released from Bicetre two years later. Another man at first ran and ran until he dropped from exhaustion; but he too recovered and was released. Chevigne, a French soldier, was unchained and over time slowly recovered his rationality and even became Pinel's trusted friend and servant. In time the doctor was able to abandon the chains and straitjackets of most of the patients and allow them freedom within the hospital.

But Pinel was frequently tested by outsiders. Men like Couthon and Robespierre often accused him of hiding enemies of the state. Once a crowd of les citoyens stormed Bicetre and surrounded Pinel, dragging him down the street to hang him from a street lamp. Suddenly Chevigne, a huge burly man, appeared and attacked the group's leaders with such fury that they fled.

In 1796 Pinel was asked to duplicate his success at Salpetriere, a former munitions arsenal which housed 8000 women patients. He acted more quickly there because of his experience at Bicetre. He freed the women, reorganized the staff, and trained personnel. There, as at Bicetre, he replaced physical treatment with what he called "moral" therapy, meaning therapy which would help patients to control their emotions. He gave them as much liberty as they could manage, but also taught them respect for authority. He set up unvarying hospital routines so that patients felt secure in their place. He also set up activities which developed the patients' abilities, such as farming on patient farms on hospital grounds. Above all, Pinel respected his patients. He saw them as people who had emotional and physical reasons for their problems. And only by careful observation could he come to understand their problems from their point of view. He did not try to speculate, but just to see what each patient saw, to understand her as a total human being so that he would understand what caused each patient to respond in different manners.

As Pinel worked with more and more patients he was able to research some of the theories concerning the cause of mental illness. One popular theory stated the cause as a deformed skull. But Pinel examined many of the patients and found that many had normal skulls. He concluded from his research that mental illness is not due to any single factor but rather to many factors, such as hereditary defects, an abnormal life, or extreme passions. In many of the cases he believed that nature could cure the disease, and so campaigned against the overuse of drugs. All of his theories and observations were included in his two major works, Traite Medico-Philoso-phique sur la Manie and Nosographique Philosophique ou Methode de L'Analyse Applique a la Medicine.

Pinel was often denounced for his ideas and methods. Many watched him carefully, pouncing whenever his treatments were unsuccessful. His reforms were first initiated in

Paris, but spread very slowly elsewhere. It was not until 1838 that the legislature tried to regulate hospital procedure and administration. And medical students received scant training in mental illness, even until the start of the twentieth century.

Despite the slow acceptance of his theories, Pinel was much honored in his later years. He held a prominent post at the Paris School of Medicine, he became Napoleon's personal physician, he was awarded the Knight of the Legion of Honor, and he was admitted to all sections of the French Academy of Sciences. However, the political changes under Louis XVIII and Charles X affected Pinel so that at the age of seventy-eight he had no position and no pension. He died after a visit to Paris and Salpetriere in 1826, neglected and penniless.

His ideas were also soon forgotten. His moral therapy was abandoned for almost a century as science progressed, growing more impersonal and materialistic. Psychological insight and sensitivity were dismissed as unscientific. Hospitals returned to a cold, distant manner of treating patients. The high recovery and discharge rates under moral therapy declined after 1860. The hope patients had felt with Pinel and his followers, like Esquirol, became despair. Again mental illness became incurable. And again interfering treatments became the popular approaches: shock treatment, drugs, baths, brain surgery. All were less successful than Pinel's approach. In fact, in 1961, the United States Joint Commission on Mental Illness and Health commented on the stagnant psychiatric health practices which needed to return to Pinel's ideas formulated in the early 1800's. Fortunately, modern-day psychiatry has returned to Pinel's more personal and hope-instilling approach to the mentally ill. And Pinel has often been honored with the title of Father of Psychiatry.

SEMMELWEIS

"The way of the world is to praise dead saints, and persecute living ones."[22]

Nathaniel Howe

In the seventeenth, eighteenth, and nineteenth centuries, as more and more people began moving into the cities, and as more charity hospitals were established for the poor, puerperal fever, a form of septicemia, became very common. Between 1652 and 1862 the disease grew to epidemic proportions two hundred times. The most serious of the epidemics killed more than 10% of the patients in lying-in hospitals. One city reported that, for more than a year, not a single hospitalized woman survived childbirth. The disease rarely appeared in homes, but rather in hospitals where hygiene was deplorable: bed linens were not changed between patients; new mothers were placed among those dying from diseases; dirty laundry sent to be cleaned came back through another door still dirty; medical students fresh from dissections examined newly delivered mothers without proper hand cleansing, etc.

The first man to wage a lifetime battle against childbed fever was the Hungarian doctor, Ignaz Philipp Semmelweis, who received his medical degree in 1844. He thereafter studied midwifery in the Lying-In Hospital in Vienna where he watched the mortality rate from puerperal fever climb to 18% in the First Clinic of the hospital. This rate was four times that of the Second Clinic, where midwives were trained. He puzzled over this high rate which appeared in only one ward of the same hospital building. He was convinced that something inside the First Clinic was causing the deaths, and he discussed various conjectures, including contagion, with other doctors. This talk soon reached his superior Professor Klein, the head obstetrician, who had written numerous articles attacking the theory of contagion. Klein was so angered by his Assistant's criticism and affrontery that he demoted

55

Semmelweis to the post of aspirant. Even Semmelweis' powerful physician friends, Hebra and Skoda, could do nothing to help him.

Soon the mortality rate in the First Clinic rose so high that the Emperor ordered an investigation. But the investigating doctors, steeped in the popular, long-held teachings of disease, concluded that the women in the First Clinic were examined more roughly by the male medical students than the women in the Second Clinic who were treated by midwives. They also stated that the women's propriety was affronted by the men who examined them, also contributing to the disease. Various other theories were propounded but Semmelweis found them all unacceptable. In 1847, the doctor who had replaced him as an assistant was offered a professorship at another university. Semmelweis was re-installed in his former post. At this time a colleague of his, Lolletschka, died suddenly of an infected scalpel wound he had received while performing an autopsy. As Semmelweis read Killetschka's autopsy report, he was struck by the similarity between his friend's symptoms and those of the women with childbed fever. He then realized that the two had the same cause: infected matter transmitted to the body through dirty hands and instruments that had touched cadavers. When he realized this, he was struck with the horror of the number of women whom he had killed. This thought haunted him all his life.

It also drove him to remedy the situation by demanding that all doctors, before examining any patients, cleanse their hands with a chlorine solution and clean sand he had placed at the clinic entrance. They were to wash with soap and water between examinations. The mortality rate fell within several months to 1.2%. Some were sure of his solution while others awaited Klein's reaction before defending or attacking the innovation. Klein opposed Semmelweis' ideas, squelching a proposal to investigate them further.

Semmelweis' students, seeing how their instructor was received, openly ridiculed the doctor and refused to cleanse their hands before examinations. The death rate began to climb again. Klein also actively worked against his assistant by withholding supplies and publicly disparaging him. Then in 1847 disaster struck. Eleven women in a row of beds died of puerperal fever. Klein now could call his assistant's prophylaxis useless. But the Hungarian doctor continued his research, discovering that infectious matter could also be transmitted from one living organism to another. He ordered that everyone wash his hands with the chlorine solution between each examination. The outcry was great. How would they ever find time to examine the patients, some jeered, with all this washing? Many refused to obey the order.

Then in 1849 Semmelweis' term of service came to an end and his application for reappointment was rejected. After several fruitless appeals, Semmelweis waited for another appointment while undertaking animal experimentation to prove his theories. Semmelweis' supporters urged him to publish the results of his work so that it would become more quickly recognized and accepted. But Semmelweis greatly disliked writing and refused to follow their suggestion. Skoda borrowed his notes and wrote up an article in his behalf which led to Semmelweis' election to the Academy of Sciences, allowing him to continue his experiments.

At last he was granted a clinical professorship by Klein but was restricted to the use of a "phantom" for teaching midwifery. Greatly insulted, Semmelweis left Vienna and returned to Budapest, discovering too late that someone had merely changed the wording of his appointment which should have included use of the cadaver as well as the phantom.

In Budapest he succeeded in gaining an excellent reputation, despite the abuse he received by other doctors. After his appointment to Professor of Obstetrics, he set to work improving the university hospital's conditions. Many resented this irascible stranger who forced them to wash their hands. Unfortunately he also angered the hospital administrator, von Tandler, when he burst into von Tandler's office with a bag of supposedly clean linens which he thrust beneath the director's nose. Such outbursts eventually led to his dismissal several years later even though the mortality rate fell to 0.39% in his first year of tenure.

In spite of the success of his innovation, noted physicians refused to accept his methods. Scanzoni, Braun, Lumpe, Virchow, and others who wrote treatises on obstetrics and puerperal fever never mentioned Semmelweis' discoveries. Until this time Semmelweis had felt that his theories would become well-known because of their great importance. But he only saw them ignored and spurned. He now began a fierce battle for recognition. In 1861 he published his first written work, <u>Die Aetiology, der Begriff und die Prophylaxis des Kindbett-fiebers</u>. In it, he said,

> Fate has chosen me as an advocate of the truths which are laid down in this work...I am constrained to come before the public...despite the many bitter hours which I have suffered, yet I find solace in the consciousness of having proposed only conclusions based upon my own convictions.[23]

With this introduction, he began his treatise which amassed the details of his life-long work in, unfortunately, a disorganized manner. He also included many bitter comments addressed to various doctors.

The book's reception was hostile and cold. This spurred Semmelweis on to write a series of open letters for which he was much criticized. They only "ran against the stone walls of professional indifference and actual hate."[24] Semmelweis began to suffer because his theories went unaccepted, and the deaths of the young mothers continued. His lectures became bitter harangues or incomprehensible monotones. Those close to him began to worry about his sanity as his behavior grew more irrational. In July of 1865, family members and friends decided to take Semmelweis to Dr. Riedel's famous sanitorium in Austria. There he was forcibly restrained by six attendants until he was put in a straitjacket and then a dark room. His wife, who was refused admittance, returned to Vienna where she fell ill. During her illness, Semmelweis died. While delivering a sick woman, he had cut a finger which became gangrenous; the infection had spread rapidly up his arm and into his chest. He died of the septicemia he had fought all his life to conquer. Twenty years later, when his doctrine was accepted by most physicians, a monument in Budapest was erected in his honor.

SMELLIE

"Such monstrous hands are, like wooden forceps, fit only to hold horses by the nose, whilst they are shod by the farrier, or stretch boots in Cranburne Alley."[25]

Elizabeth Nihell

William Smellie (1697-1763), born in Lanark, Scotland, probably entered the medical profession by apprenticeship. References in his treatise to his early experiences show that he was from the outset very interested in midwifery. He successfully practiced medicine in Lanark for nineteen years, during this time becoming a member of the Faculty of Physicians and Surgeons of Glasgow—a corporation which controlled medical practice in western Scotland. In 1739 he gave up his practice in Lanark and after traveling to Europe to practice with the most well-known European doctors, settled in London where he practiced and taught midwifery. Smellie wished to promote and improve this branch of medicine which by this time interested him exclusively.

His early progress in London was in no way remarkable. He was a foreigner and he lacked the social graces needed to advance rapidly in London. But he began to teach and to attract many students interested in midwifery—a branch of medicine still largely closed to men. His course consisted of lectures with demonstrations on an ingenuous machine he had invented. It consisted of a skeletal female pelvis and lower abdomen covered with layers of imitation muscle and skin. It was constructed so that the uterus could be contracted or dilated as in childbirth. Toy fetuses accompanied the machine. Their limbs were maneuverable and the cranium, elastic. Smellie used these fetuses to demonstrate progressive fetal positions and the various presentations at delivery.

But Smellie realized that the course was inadequate without clinical teaching. He therefore advertised to the poor sections of London that he with his students would attend poor women in their homes at the time of their delivery at no cost. He also set up a fund to help the needier women. Usually only three or four students attended, but Smellie recorded one case in which twenty-eight crowded into the room to observe the delivery. Alarmed by this great number, a threatening mob formed outside and only dispersed when they were told that both the mother and child were alive and safe.

It was unusual and generally unacceptable for a women to be attended by a male accoucheur, and unthinkable by twenty-eight male observers. Midwives still dominated this field, although to qualify for their profession they needed only an endorsement from some established midwife, a small fee, and an oath not to practice witchcraft. Consequently, childbed mishaps were frequent and horrendous. Gradually the monopoly was beginning to slacken as medicine finally moved beyond traditional Galenian authority. This allowed independent thinkers like Smellie to improve child-birthing techniques. Another reason was the introduction of forceps which called for more knowledge and skill than the majority of midwives had. It was already fashionable on the Continent for upper class women to be accompanied by man-midwives after Louis XIV employed Jules Clement to attend his mistress during her delivery. For all these reasons and perhaps also because more and more people were uneasy about the poor training most midwives had, men were slowly gaining acceptance.

Smellie made a very positive contribution to this movement to improve lying-in conditions for poor women and education for both midwives and medical students. But since he was one of the first in this movement, he also had to fight the many prejudices against men in midwifery. First, some of his patients had difficulty accepting him. One woman screamed, "Murder!" when he attempted to examine her. And as no respectable woman would expose her body to a man, he had to operate under the sheets which sometimes caused inadvertent errors. Smellie's person and manners also caused problems. He was a huge man with very large hands which his detractors particularly liked to ridicule. His dress, although well-intentioned, was also odd. He believed that his attire should be feminized to make him more acceptable to women. He thus wore a loose nightgown, a waistcoat without arms and a shirt with pinned up sleeves. To this he added a bonnet which would cover his wig. His baiters had endless sport with this getup, especially Mrs. Nihell, the leading London midwife, who called him a "great-horse-god-mother of a he-midwife."[26]

During these early years of teaching, Smellie realized that his professional standing could be improved if he acquired his Doctorate of Medicine degree. This was granted him in 1745. But this degree and his growing reputation as an excellent man-midwife never helped him to acquire a practice among the upper classes. But he did more than any other individual to advance obstetrics in the 1700's.

His teachings can be found in his three-volume <u>Treatise on The Theory and Practice of Midwifery</u>. In this treatise can be found the first description of the positions of the fetus before birth. Every other physician had assumed that the fetus lay with its head toward the top and after the seventh month, tumbled over so that it was in a crawling position on its hands and knees. So here Smellie exploded an idea held since the time of Hippocrates. He also gave the first clear description of the movement of the head in relation to the pelvis during birth. Smellie, also for the first time, completely described the mechanism of labor. Another idea he went on to demolish was the misunderstanding that the cervix closed immediately after childbirth. This made the removal of the placenta a great concern. Many removed the placenta manually. Others believed in pulling the cord. Smellie, however, was willing to allow Nature a chance first.

The area in which Smellie caused the greatest furor was his use of forceps. Smellie had designed a pair of short, light forceps shaped to the pelvic curve and wrapped in leather for

63

cushioning. The wrappings were changed after each use. In his teachings he was very careful to clarify when forceps were to be used. He himself said he used them only when absolutely necessary and even then in only ten out of a thousand deliveries. But many, not understanding or even knowing his teachings or his practice, accused him of abusing the use of forceps.

These accusations began early in his London teaching career. The 1700's were the age of the pamphleteer and the lampooner. And Smellie became the butt and object of their personal attacks. The midwives furiously attacked him and his use of forceps through Mrs. Nihell's shrill writings. Another person, Dr. William Douglas, could not endure Smellie's growing reputation and wrote scathing attacks in order to besmirch it. Philip Thicknesse, a fashionable quack, pretended to be horrified at Smellie's descriptions of vaginal examinations and in several pamphlets branded the Scotsman's treatise as indecent and shameful. The most bitter attack came from Dr. John Burton, a well-educated and prosperous man who founded York Hospital. Burton considered himself the expert on childbirth. He, too, had designed a pair of forceps modeled on the principle of a lobster's claw. He had published an essay of his theories and practices which had received an unfavorable notice. Smellie's treatise appeared shortly thereafter and was praised. In a 233-page letter to Smellie, Burton condemns every facet of the Scotsman's teachings and practices. Perhaps in a case of poetic justice, Burton gained immortality as the original Dr. Slopin in Laurence Sterne's Tristram Shandy. Smellie ignored these attacks. Only once did he answer an attack and that was in a letter to a student. Otherwise he did nothing.

Smellie's London life ended in 1759. He had, in nineteen years in the capital, taught 900 students, a number of them famous men, such as William Hunter, and some women. He had endured many attacks and accusations, only once troubling to refute them. At the age of sixty-two, asthma forced him to retire. In 1759 he returned to Lanark where he completed the third volume of his treatise. He sent it to his friend, Tobias Smollet, for editing, but did not live to see it in print.

Smellie was not a genius, but he was a great physician and scientist because he could cast aside authority, tradition, and superstition to think for himself. He could see things as they are, not as they had been described centuries before. In this way he cleared away the rubbish that had surrounded midwifery. He taught a reasoned trust in the natural progress of labor under normal conditions; he then taught the handling of difficult labors. In this he can easily be called the father of obstetrics. And yet he was forgotten at the time of his death. It was 130 years after his death before a worthy biography was published in England. Perhaps this time was needed to forget that Smellie never attended a "lady," and to realize that Smellie did not advocate the use of forceps except in special circumstances with many precautions; and to see the magnitude of his work in perspective.

SYDENHAM

"It is my nature to think where others read, to ask, less whether the world agrees with me than whether I agree with the truth, and to hold cheap the rumour and applause of the multitude."[27]

Thomas Sydenham

Thomas Sydenham (1624-1689) had been in medical school at Oxford only two months when England was thrown into civil war by the King's Cavaliers and the Parliament's Roundheads. Sydenham fought in the Parliamentary Army, a political choice which affected his career, taken up after the end of the Royalist resistance. He received his Bachelor of Medicine, a belated military honor granted him because of his support of Cromwell. He then went on to All Souls' College where he spent several years as a fellow and then as senior bursar. During these years, he became acquainted with Robert Boyle, who kindled his interest in epidemic diseases. But the young doctor was still too involved with politics to devote all his energy to medicine.

With Cromwell's death and the Restoration, Sydenham went abroad for several months. His name, once an asset, was now a liability. He had previously been allowed to practice medicine without a proper license. But after he returned from France, he was obligated to take examinations in order to be granted a licentiate from the College of Physicians. Because he could no longer give his time to political interests, he now concerned himself solely with medicine, although the taint of his previous political affiliations never left him.

Now fully involved in medicine, he displayed his greatest merit as a physician and scientist—his ability to avoid the popular and traditional medical beliefs. He avoided both Galenic orthodoxy and the new speculative medicine. He called for a renewal of the empirical approach to medicine. And in so doing he re-established Hippocrates' basic principle which called for close observation of disease.

He decided to set down accurately what he observed without allowing various theories to sway his observations. Then he would learn to recognize specific diseases. Sydenham revolutionized clinical medicine by basing his treatment on careful observation rather than on Galenic dogma or on speculative theory. He began a careful compilation of his work which was rewritten several times and eventually published as Observationes Medicae (1676). In this work, Sydenham classified and described the fevers prevalent in London between 1661 and 1675. All the fevers were placed in one of three categories: "continued" diseases, such as typhus and typhoid; "intermittent," such as malaria; and smallpox. After careful classification, he suggested the most efficacious methods of treating these diseases. Many of his unorthodox ideas met with disdain, some rightfully so.

His theories concerning smallpox caused a major controversy. The accepted treatment for this scourge was a heating treatment that included heating cordials and heavy, suffocating blankets. Sydenham prescribed a more moderate regimen that called for patients to be kept out of bed as long as possible and when in bed, covered with just the usual bedclothes. He was quite successful with this procedure. Unfortunately, his success led him to theorize incorrectly as to the cause of smallpox, and his erroneous theory caused doctors to reject both his theory and his treatment, which was much more effective than their own. Sydenham later discarded his theory that smallpox was a natural process in life and thus should be tampered with as little as possible, but not before stirring up great antagonism because of his blunt statements blaming the high mortality rate on meddlesome physicians. He also claimed that a strong, healthy man would succumb if he were subjected to the popular treatments given the sick. Small wonder that so many sick died, he said.

The physicians were infuriated. One doctor, remembering Sydenham's political activities, called him a "trooper turned physician," "a Western bumpkin that pretends to Limbo children in the Small-pox by a new method," and "this generalissimo."[28] Some of his detractors also considered withdrawing his license because of his irregular practice. Sydenham himself said, "What stories of extravagancy and folly have the talk of prejudiced people brought upon me, so much that it has been told to persons of quality that I have taken those who have had the small pox out of their beds and put them in cold water."[29]

These sorts of controversies which dogged him all his life harmed his reputation in higher medical circles. He was never elected to the Royal College of Physicians because of his unacceptable medical practices and because of his previous political connections. His poor reputation affected him in other ways, too. Sometimes when doctors wished to consult with him, they felt obliged to do so secretly.

Despite his problems with those in higher medical circles, Sydenham gained an excellent reputation with the public and with some of the younger, more open-minded doctors who agreed with his empirical principles. Sydenham grew famous because of his histories of fevers and other conditions. He described pleurisy, pneumonia, rheumatism, scarlet fever, gout, renal calculus, and many others. He developed a systematic account of diseases, especially of fevers, where none had existed before. He has, thus, been called the forerunner of the science of epidemiology: In addition, he wrote about psychological medicine, describing hysteria, psychosis, and hypochondriasis, although he did not differentiate between them.

Sydenham's innovative treatments also brought him fame. He advanced several useful remedies. He showed that insufficient iron is sometimes the cause of anemia. He realized the value of laudanum for those in great pain. He also discovered that quinine cures malaria. And he recommended peruvian bark for agues, although an opportunist stole his idea and became a wealthy man through this venture. But, perhaps most important of all, he often dispensed with drugs altogether, and prescribed daily exercise, fresh air, a wholesome and moderate diet, and mineral waters. This was probably his most innovative treatment in an age when drugs were regularly and overly prescribed.

Patients as well as doctors refused his prescription of fresh air and exercise because it did not smack of proper medicine. A story is sometimes told of a patient who refused this remedy. So Sydenham told him that he could do no more for him and referred him to a doctor in a distant town. The patient rode horseback to reach the town only to find that no doctor of that name had ever existed in the town. Indignant and angry, he returned to discover that Sydenham had deceived him into getting fresh air and exercise and that he was also feeling much better.

As physicians throughout Europe began to see the usefulness of his Hippocratic principle of observation and of his successful remedies, his opinions were soon highly valued and carried great authority. And although he always had his detractors, he also gained a group of loyal supporters who saw that he had pointed out a method for advancing clinical medicine based on observation and experience. Upon his death, the College of Physicians erected a tablet in his honor which bears these words: "A Physician Famous for All Time."

TAGLIACOZZI

"But this much I can honestly assert, that I have not omitted or suppressed anything pertaining to the subject. For this I should like to receive credit and to be blamed by none, for it would ill befit any worthy or honest man to criticize. And if there are some whom these fruits of my labor may help, I freely grant them the use thereof. As for others, I earnestly request that they treat this work not with scorn or ridicule, but benevolently."[30]

Gaspare Tagliacozzi

Many believe that plastic surgery originated during World War I. But the earliest record of plastic surgery can be dated to 400 A.D. in India. This manuscript is only a copy, however, of a much older text which some experts believe was originally written down around 600 B.C. Even then the surgery was probably ancient. The Hindu method of nose repair was especially prevalent because amputation of the nose was a common punishment for various crimes. The earliest European writer to discuss plastic surgery was the Roman Celsus who lived from 25 B.C. to 50 A.D. Then, much mention of plastic surgery appears in the fourteenth and fifteenth century medical literature. During this time Antonio Branca developed the Italian method of rhinoplasty, using the reparative flap from the arm. But only reports of his works remain. These reports occasionally erred. Falloppio's treatise, for example, stated that the graft was taken from the arm's muscle. In fact, he said, a hole was dug in the arm and the nose placed in the hole. He claimed that the process would take up to a year and involve great torment. His authoritative discussion tended to discredit the whole technique.

Despite this discreditation, patients still demanded plastic surgery. Frequent duels and brawls, sword clashes, constant wars, family vendettas—all made the loss of ears, lips, and nose common. Noblemen and wealthy merchants were willing to endure pain and high fees to have their mutilated faces repaired.

Gaspare Tagliacozzi, who held his doctorate in both medicine and philosophy as was customary, saw a great need for good plastic surgeons, especially in a time when the whole subject was shot through with erroneous concepts and prejudices. Tagliacozzi was taught by Giulio Arnazio, a Balognese professor who imparted to his students various methods of plastic surgery. Tagliacozzi then began experiments which led him to perfect these methods, particularly the nose repair. He lifted up a flap of flesh from the forearm and, after fourteen days, applied it to the nose which had been scarified. The arm was then bound to the face. After four or five days, the lap of skin was usually attached to the nose. The forearm end was cut away and the flap trimmed and shaped to fit the nose.

A prominent physician and anatomist, Mercuriale, had heard of Tagliacozzi's techniques and praised him in his treatise. Tagliacozzi, reading the encouraging words, decided the time had come to rectify the common misconceptions about nose repair. In a letter to Mercuriale, he explained the principles of nose reconstructions and corrected the often repeated errors. This letter was published in the second edition of Mercuriale's treatise.

With this publication and with his many successful surgeries, Tagliacozzi's fame began to grow. His position as professor at the University of Balogna improved as he was given more pay and more prestigious responsibilities. Many of his patients now were of high birth. He was associated with the leading princes in Italy who continually consulted him.

In 1597, Tagliacozzi published his De Curtorum Chirurgia per Insitionem, which he had been preparing for almost fifteen years. In this volume, which contained numerous illustrations, he discussed many methods of plastic surgery. He then described his own and explained why he thought them the most effective. The treatise had a mixed reception. Some felt it wrong to tinker with the body God had given man. Others could not escape their preconceptions and continued to believe the errors passed on by other doctors. Others applauded it as the first work to organize plastic surgery on a scientific basis.

Tagliacozzi, however, did not live long enough to see the final outcome. He died in 1599. It was after his death that Tagliacozzi's reputation was attacked. During his lifetime he had come to great fame. But shortly after his death, his reputation and character were defamed. Rumors were spread that Tagliacozzi's remarkable successes were the result of magic. Soon nuns in the church where he was buried claimed that they heard a voice condemning Tagliacozzi. Physicians and clergymen were, regrettably, trapped in superstition as was everyone else, and the doctor's body was ordered exhumed and moved to unconsecrated ground. Four years later, Tagliacozzi's honor and innocence were proven and his body was reburied in consecrated ground.

Tagliacozzi's theories and methods, however, fell into disgrace. Misconceptions Tagliacozzi had worked so hard to obliterate took hold again. Those who had been envious of the doctor's stature but too awed by his rank to trouble him, began to spread rumors. And although his friends and supporters had demanded an investigation that cleared him of all charges, the blow to Tagliacozzi's reputation had damaged his credibility beyond repair. It is interesting to note that one of his denouncers was Girolamo Sbaragli, the same man who had so mistreated Marcello Malpighi. Malpighi respected Tagliacozzi's progressive methods. And Sbaragli attacked Tagliacozzi's reputation in another effort to discredit Malpighi.

Plastic surgery, particularly rhinoplasty, fell into disuse soon after Tagliacozzi's death. It was neglected for almost two centuries. Occasionally physicians discovered his treatise and wished to revive his methods, but to no avail. Many false beliefs surrounded the procedures. People incorrectly believed that the flap of skin used for nose repair was taken

73

from another person. Then because they were superstitious, they thought that when the donor died, the reconstructed nose would also die because of sympathy between the two. For these and many other reasons the Paris Faculty interdicted face reconstruction altogether.

Tagliacozzi was soon considered a buffoon whose methods were often ridiculed in popular plays and poetry. Samuel Butler, Addison and Steele, and William Congreve all mocked the idea of the sympathetic nose. Perhaps Butler's ridicule in Hudibras is the most comic. A porter has donated part of his derriere to make a new nose for his employer. But when the porter dies, the donated nose drops off. Tagliacozzi and his techniques were ridiculed in this manner for many years. And yet he had been loved by his students and respected by his colleagues and patients, the leading men of his day. Fortunately, the revival of interest in plastic surgery also brought his work to light. And he can now be once again accorded the honor and respect due him as an innovative and skilled plastic surgeon.

VESALIUS

"Great men...men who struggle alone for a great
cause, are like great rivers. Debris may block their
waters, but it never stops them from flowing."[31]

Felix Marti-Ibanez

Andreas Vesalius, born in 1514 in Brussels, Belgium,
studied medicine in Paris under Sylvius, the well-known
anatomist. Sylvius taught and conducted the dissections of the
human body from a podium removed from the dissection
table. As he would read from one of Galen's texts, someone
else would dissect the body. And whatever was dissected was
made to conform to Galen's sketches and descriptions. Vesalius
disliked this manner of instruction. He began to dissect bodies
himself, discovering that some of Galen's teachings were
incorrect. But he knew he had to thoroughly investigate these
discrepancies before he could announce his discoveries.

When he was twenty-four, he accepted the position of
professor of anatomy in Padua, Italy, where he was respected
as an anatomist. He was able to dissect more often because he
had greater access to bodies in Padua than in Paris, although
obtaining them was still difficult. Vesalius was often forced
to get his bodies illegally. Once he even approached the
criminal court justices, asking them to order executions at
times suitable to his teaching schedule and to order executions
that were less mutilating. But dissection was still banned by
the church, and the outcome of Vesalius' direct appeals is not
known.

As Vesalius carried on his investigations he found more
and more contradictions with Galen's texts. He decided to
publish his own anatomy text. In 1543, when Vesalius was
only twenty-eight, he traveled to Basel, Switzerland, where he
published his treatise, De Humanis Corporis Fabrica. Vesalius
was immediately and fiercely attacked. Many scientists
turned against him. His former instructor, Sylvius, led the

75

attack. How could Vesalius contradict Galen, he asked. Even if Vesalius were correct, he said, sixteenth century man's anatomy was probably very different from Galen's second century man's anatomy. Either that or copyists had made errors over the fourteen centuries of copying Galen's teachings. But Galen himself could not be wrong. Vesalius, or, as Sylvius called him veranus, which means "donkey," and his followers, whom he called two-legged asses, were certainly wrong. Others joined in the attack.

When Vesalius returned to Padua, seeking quiet in the storm that had hit him, he found that his students and fellow-professors had turned against him. A favorite student, Realdo Columbus, had undermined his authority and had discredited him in order to secure his position as professor of anatomy in Padua. Then Vesalius was asked to leave Padua, perhaps at the Emperor's request. He was preparing to go to the court of the Hapsburg emperor, Charles V, in Brussels, Belgium, when news reached him that the Flemish court physicians were trying to discredit him before his arrival, saying that he knew little about medical science or medical practice. The treachery of Columbus, the intrigue of the court physicians, the attacks on his treatise—all so embittered and angered Vesalius that he gathered and burned all his notebooks and manuscripts. In 1544, he left for Brussels never to return to Padua.

Vesalius served Charles V until the Emperor abdicated his throne to his son. During Charles V's reign, Vesalius was able to edit and publish a second edition to his text. In this edition, he was careful to remove any information that might entangle him with the Inquisition. He removed his remarks about the greed and immorality of the clergy and clarified various statements about dissection. Vesalius' work with anatomy did not cease with the burning of his writings.

After Charles V abdicated, Vesalius became court physician for Philip II. In 1559 he followed Philip II to Madrid, Spain. By this time his contributions to anatomy were beginning to receive notice. Occasionally his text was quoted and scientific publications were dedicated to him. Despite this encouraging turn, Vesalius did not prosper in Spain. The Spanish, who attacked the Moors and the Jews, also disliked the Flemish. His Spanish rivals scrutinized his work and informed the Emperor that Vesalius was incompetent. But he was too prominent a courtier to dispose of easily. So the Spanish waited and watched.

One day Vesalius received a summons to the Holy Inquisition. Different versions of the reason appear in histories today. But one plausible version states that an important courtier died and his family allowed Vesalius to perform an autopsy, although they feared that the courtier might only be in a trance. When Vesalius opened the chest, an observer claimed that he saw the heart still beating. Vesalius was charged with murder. The Inquisition wanted to execute him but Philip II intervened and the death sentence was dropped. Instead Vesalius was compelled to make a pilgrimage to Jerusalem. He died in 1564 while returning from the Holy Land after he was shipwrecked on the island of Zante.

Although Vesalius' work did not receive the attention it deserved during his lifetime, it would become slowly accepted. Over the next two centuries, twenty-five more editions of his text were issued throughout Europe. Vesalius had opened another "breach in the fortress of Galenism."[32]

WELLS

"My husband's great gift which he devoted to the service of mankind proved a curse to himself and to his family."[33]

Mrs. Horace Wells

In 1844, a dentist, Horace Wells, witnessed an exhibition of the amusing effects of nitrous oxide. The exhibitor, Gardner Quincy Colton, had arranged a private demonstration for those who showed special interest in "laughing gas." One of the volunteers, Samuel Cooley, who worked in a local drugstore, inhaled the gas and soon burst into hilarious antics. An assistant from a rival drugstore started guffawing at Cooley, who suddenly became angry and chased his rival, crashing into benches and knocking them over. Wells watched the scene puzzled rather than amused for he saw that Cooley had struck himself severely several times and did not appear to have noticed it. Later he asked Cooley if he was not hurt. Cooley pulled up his trouser-legs and saw, to his amazement, that he had some severe bruises and cuts which he did not recollect receiving.

Wells was excited about this discovery because he was certain that the nitrous oxide had deadened any sensation of pain. What an important development for dentistry! The very next day he asked Colton to help him with an experiment. Colton hesitated because he was not sure how safe or powerful the gas was. Wells said that he would have one of his own teeth extracted while inhaling the gas, and that would settle the argument.

And so Wells, Colton, and two dentists assembled in the surgical room. Colton gave the gasbag to Wells who began to inhale the nitrous oxide slowly and regularly. His face turned ashen and his lips blue. The attending dentist, Riggs, immediately pulled the tooth. When he released Wells' head, it fell forward on his chest. The men were frightened. Was he dead?

79

They looked at each other and then stared at Wells' face. Suddenly Wells began to move. He opened his mouth and his eyes and, seeing the tooth just extracted, was so startled that he exclaimed, "A new era in tooth-pulling!"[34] And then he went on to say how he had not felt even a pin's prick.

An impetuous man who was easily excited, Wells was immediately ready to open up a practice advertising painless extractions, but his friends cautioned him to learn more about the gas's safety and efficacy and insisted that he get someone of good scientific standing to support his claim. Wells knew a chemistry professor, Charles Jackson, who had once given him a certificate of approval for a dental solder he had developed which would not corrode. Wells took a previous partner, William Morton, with him to see Jackson. The chemist listened condescendingly to the story of the painless tooth extraction. Then he ordered Wells to abandon his crazy experiments. Man would never overcome pain; scientists knew pain was inevitable and mere dentists had no place questioning established scientific beliefs.

Wells was furious with Jackson and decided to embarrass him by taking his discovery to the prestigious John Collins Warren of the Massachusetts General Hospital. But Wells had not experimented adequately with nitrous oxide to know correct dosages or the various effects of the gas on different individuals. So when he entered the room to demonstrate his discovery, he was not well prepared. One of the Harvard medical students who had a bad tooth volunteered to be the guinea-pig and sat waiting in the chair. Wells was so excited and nervous that he was fumbling and dropping instruments. But at last he gave the student the gas. Then he clamped his forceps down on the tooth and began to pull. The student let out a terrified scream and all the observers began to laugh and boo, shouting that the whole affair was "humbug." Wells fled from the room. A later interrogation of the patient proved that despite his scream, he had felt no pain. But Wells had been publicly embarrassed.

80

He attempted one last demonstration in his hometown but gave the patient too much gas, almost killing him. With this second defeat he decided to give up dentistry. He gave up his practice and rented his house. As quickly as he had taken up his interest with nitrous oxide, he now dropped it. He had been quick to recognize an important potential use for nitrous oxide, but he did not have the endurance to work out the problems involved with the gas.

And so he left dentistry. For a while he worked as a historian, then as a traveling bird fancier with a troup of singing canaries, then as a salesman of shower-baths and coal-sifters, and at last as a dealer in old paintings and engravings. He continued with this erratic lifestyle, always an imaginative, creative man who for some reason lacked the ability to carry out his dreams.

While in Paris buying a shipment of paintings, Wells read news of the discovery of anesthesia by William Morton and a possible reward of $100,000 for the discoverer. He thought that although Morton was using ether, he, Wells, had discovered the idea of inducing temporary unconsciousness by inhaling gas. He lodged a protest with the Academy of Science and returned to America ready for acclaim. Instead he was cold-shouldered and ignored. In indignation he tried to assert his claim, but made no headway. An official investigation called to settle the battle between the claimants for the discovery of anesthesia excluded his claim because he had not worked with ether.

Wells then set out to discredit Morton by finding a gas superior to ether. He began experimenting with chloroform and tried to persuade doctors and dentists to use this gas, but they were satisfied with ether and just ignored him. By this time, in desperation, he was using chloroform himself and was addicted to it. His health, both physical and mental, was soon undermined.

He frequented New York dives and brothels, thinking the people in these places were the only ones who now would accept him. But soon even the prostitutes grew tired of him and ignored him. In rage at this final rejection and under the influence of chloroform, he threw a vial of vitriolic acid in a prostitute's face. He was immediately arrested and the New York Evening Post carried an account of this "diabolical outrage."[35] Two days later in the Tombs Prison, Horace Wells committed suicide, lacerating his left thigh to the bone, severing the femoral artery. In his cell were found three letters, one to his wife, another to a solicitor, and the third to a newspaper. He explained his suicide: "My character, which I have ever prized above everything else, is gone. My dear, dear wife and child, how they will suffer. I cannot proceed. My brain is on fire."[36]

Less than one hundred years later, Wells was recognized for his role in the development of anesthesia. His discovery helped to bring freedom from pain to humankind but only stark tragedy to himself and his family.

WRIGHT

"Two staffs are necessary in a hospital—one to
teach all that is known, the other to teach that we
know nothing—and to get on with it."[37]

Almroth Wright

In a collection of bicentennial essays entitled Advances in
American Medicine, the only reference to Almroth Wright
under the heading of the history of immunology is one
negative sentence stating that Wright discouraged Fleming
from studying penicillin because he believed that what harmed
bacteria could harm man; the only correct approach was to
strengthen the patient's defenses. One negative comment
about a man whose work tremendously advanced the field of
immunology.

Almroth Wright was born in Ireland, where he began his
life-long medical studies. As he was a brilliant student, he
won a traveling scholarship to Leipzig where he started his
apprenticeship in medical research. In Germany he was
introduced to many new technical devices, some of which he
later adopted for his own use, others which he designed for
himself. He was also introduced to many developments in
medical knowledge and decided to devote his life to medical
scientific work. But starting in this field was difficult, especially financially.

For a while he read law, winning a studentship. When the
studentship money was exhausted, he entered the Civil Service. Then he accepted a demonstratorship at Cambridge.
Another scholarship allowed him to return to Germany. Then
he traveled to the University of Sydney where he was offered
a demonstratorship. He returned to England where he finally
found a more permanent niche as chairman of pathology at the
Army Medical School. He taught pathology and bacteriology
three mornings a week for eight months. The rest of his time
was free for research.

He immediately began to study blood coagulation and microbic disease. He wanted to make the diagnosis of microbic disease more exact. This exactness would make it possible to prevent some of these diseases (Pasteur had already made a tremendous start with anthrax of sheep and chicken cholera). He had also read Metchnikoff's observations on the removal of foreign bodies by the phagocytes of insects. He saw that the extension of these observations might help him to understand how man recovers from infection. They might also suggest how to assist their recovery. All these dreams Wright helped to achieve over the next fifty years.

The first disease he targeted was Malta fever. Evidence showed that protection could be obtained both by living and killed vaccine, that there was little difference between the two. To test this assertion, Wright injected himself with first the killed vaccine and second the living culture. But the protection was inadequate and he was ill for several weeks. However, during his recovery he was already busy with a far more serious problem, typhoid.

In 1895 the word "typhoid" was like a curse for it brought death to more than 5,000 people a year in England and to more than 35,000 people a year in the USA. Of course, many more recovered from prolonged illness. The death rate was ten to thirty percent of those who contracted the disease. Wright saw that proper sanitation had greatly reduced the death rate, but he still saw the need for medical intervention, especially in case of war when sanitation systems would most certainly break down. The Germans attributed more than sixty percent of the deaths of their troops in the Franco-Prussian War to typhoid.

Wright began testing his blood and the blood of volunteers who allowed themselves to be inoculated. He found that a normal man's blood could kill a few typhoid microbes; but after inoculation it could kill ten to fifty times as many. This extra killing power usually remained for quite some time after the inoculation. He also recognized a short phase of lessened

84

killing power after inoculation when the patient might be somewhat ill. For the person who already harbored typhoid bacilli this could be dangerous, so he advised that vaccine doses be no larger than necessary. And the inoculated person was to be observed for several days. Later many disregarded these precautions and this worked against the general acceptance of the vaccine.

Wright now needed to have his vaccine tested on a large scale, logically in the Army. But widespread inoculation was too novel an idea, Wright too young a man, and his ideas too unorthodox. Besides, he had been appointed to his post over the head of an officer who expected the promotion. This officer actively opposed Wright's work. But, Wright continued his fight. The vaccine was tried in various parts of the world over the next five years. Results with troops in India were so favorable that the procedure was sanctioned there. Four percent of the troops going to the Boer War in South Africa were inoculated. But it was almost impossible to follow them. So statistics were not very helpful. And, in fact, statistics became the center of a serious conflict. Wright was prepared to act on probability. But other physicians and scientists claimed the vaccine protection was too irregular.

The War Office Committee decided on a compromise. For three years, inoculations were to be given with proper precautions and then careful records were to be kept for all troops going abroad. But the inoculations were still on a volunteer basis. When World War I broke out in 1914, Wright offered his lab to Lord Kitchener for high-speed production of vaccine. He than published an open letter to The Times which explained the problem. Lord Kitchener then decreed that no man would be sent overseas unless first inoculated. By the end of 1915 almost all of the British Expeditionary Force was immunized. Wright's battle had begun in 1897—almost two decades spent fighting for typhoid immunization.

Wright left the Army Medical Service with whom relations had always been uneasy and became the pathologist at

St. Mary's Hospital. After openly discussing the inadequate salary and provisions for medical research there, he was off to a difficult start there as well. He displeased the hierarchy with his frankness about medical affairs. But he found a kindred soul in Captain Stewart Rankin Douglas. The two men began to study phagocytosis in the living human body. They discovered that Metchnikoff's description of the disposal of microbes was too simple. Before the phagocytes engulfed and digested the foreign bodies, the microbes had to be somehow prepared. This was done by a property of the blood serum which Wright named "opsonic." This discovery was of great importance. It clarified our understanding of the recovery mechanism; it gave us a precision method of diagnosing some microbic diseases; and it opened up a new field for the treatment of these diseases.

But this discovery was greatly opposed by the medical hierarchy who were not prepared to put these new discoveries into practice. Once again, statistics became the point of contention.

Wright went on with his work, investigating wound infection. He brought out two important points: that microbes differ in their growth ability in blood fluids; that the inability of many microbes to grow in blood fluids depends on the antitryptic principle in the blood. These were far-reaching discoveries that even by the 1950's had not been adopted into medical science. Bacteriologists for years paid little heed to these aspects of infection.

Why was Wright so often either opposed or ignored? The medical world was never too interested in his work. Gradually the number of his students waned, audiences at his public lectures decreased, and visitors at his lab were fewer and fewer. There were several reasons for this. First, his influence lessened over the years as he bluntly stated his unconventional ideas. He disliked reticence and saw no reason for suppressing any of his thoughts. But his combativeness antagonized physicians and scientists in many quarters. He had also acquired a reputation summarized in a name given him, Sir Almost Wright. Others disliked the fact that his laboratory sold vaccines to pharmacies. They seldom questioned his integrity, but claimed this practice could fetter scientific freedom. Scientists also looked askance at his technical methods of research which were often in their developmental stages. But Wright was also plagued by a problem that always meets innovators: They are rarely given a warm welcome. Many people do not welcome any disturbance to their views. And so it was with Wright and his ideas, for instance, his contention that antiseptics in infected wounds often do no good.

But these reasons seem too small to have caused such a great neglect of his work. Much of his work he embodied in his Creed which contains nineteen items. These were forgotten through the indifference of the medical world. Only one was proven wrong in his lifetime, as Wright acknowledged, and yet the others were not studied or further researched. They were simply laid aside.

Wright continued his work, seeing many improvements to the research facilities at St. Mary's. At the age of eighty-four he gave up regular visits to the lab. In 1946 he resigned as Head of the Inoculation Department, a position he had held since its inception thirty-eight years before. He died at the age of eighty-six.

POSTSCRIPT

What can we learn from these almost unbelievable vignettes of real life?

We learn that Machiavelli, the great master of intrigue, was perhaps right when he said "one half of one percent of the people learn from the experience of others, two and one half percent learn from their own experience and the remaining ninety-seven percent never learn from the experience of others or from their own experiences."

It is my strong hope that you, the reader, are among the three percent. For, we are told that those of us who can't learn from the history or others are doomed to repeat their mistakes.

CHRONOLOGICAL LIST

Gerolamo Cardano	1501-1576
Ambroise Paré	c.1510-1590
Andreas Vesalius	1514-1564
Gaspare Tagliacozzi	1545-1599
Thomas Sydenham	1624-1689
Marcello Malpighi	1628-1694
William Smellie	1697-1763
James Lind	1716-1794
John Hunter	1728-1793
John Morgan	1735-1789
Philippe Pinel	1745-1826
John Elliotson	1791-1868
Harriot Hunt	1805-1875
Horace Wells	1815-1847
Ignaz Semmelweis	1818-1865
William Hammond	1828-1900
Almroth Wright	1861-1947

FOOTNOTES

1. Oystein Ore, Cardano, the Gambling Scholar (Princeton: Princeton University Press, 1953), pp. 12-13.
2. Alan Wykes, Doctor Cardano, Physician Extraordinary (London: Muller, 1969), pp. 71-72.
3. Ore, p. 52.
4. Andre Gide quoted in The Shorter Bartlett's Familiar Quotations, ed. Christopher Morley (New York: Permabooks, 1953), p. 140.
5. Robin McKnown, Pioneers in Mental Health (New York: Dodd, Mead, 1961), pp. 120-121.
6. James Gregory Mumford, A Narrative of Medicine in America (Philadelphia: Lippincott, 1903), pp. 46-47.
7. Harriot Kezia Hunt quoted in Mary Roth Walsh, Doctors Wanted: No Women Need Apply (New Haven: Yale University Press, 1977), pp. 28-29.
8. The National Cyclopedia of American Biography (New York: J. T. White and Co., 1899), 9, p. 259.
9. The National Cyclopedia, p. 259.
10. John Hunter, letter to William Hunter, quoted in Sarah Regal Reidman, Masters of the Scalpel: the Story of Surgery (Chicago: Rand MacNally, 1962), pp. 101-102.
11. John Hunter, quoted in John Kobler, The Reluctant Surgeon: a Biography of John Hunter (Garden City, N. Y.: Doubleday, 1960), pp. 164-165.
12. Kobler, pp. 164-165.
13. Sir John Simon, quoted in M. E. M. Walker, Pioneers of Public Health: the Story of Some Benefactors of the Human Race (rpt. 1930; Freeport, N. Y.: Books for Libraries Press, 1968), pp. 23-24.
14. Herbert Spencer quoted in Louis Harry Roddis, James Lind: Founder of Nautical Medicine (New York: Schuman, 1950), pp. 73-74.
15. Marcello Malpighi quoted by Tibor Doby, Discoverers

of Blood Circulation (London: Abelard-Schuman, 1963), p. 244.

16. John Morgan quoted in James Thomas Flexner, Doctors on Horseback: Pioneers of American Medicine (New York: Viking Press, 1937), p. 48.

17. Flexner, pp. 16-18.

18. John E. Keiffer, "Philadelphia Controversy, 1775-1780," The Bulletin of the History of Medicine, 11 (1942), pp. 152-154.

19. Caleb C. Colton, The New Dictionary of Thoughts, comp. Tyrone Edwards (New York: Doubleday, 1955), p. 178.

20. Kenneth Walker, Story of Medicine (New York: Oxford University Press, 1955), pp. 112-113.

21. Philip S. Callahan, Tuning in to Nature (Old Greenwich, Conn.: The Devin-Adair Co., 1975), p. 40.

22. Nathaniel Howe quoted in The New Dictionary of Thoughts, comp. Tyrone Edwards (New York: Doubleday, 1955), p. 396.

23. Ignaz Philipp Semmelweis, The Cause, Concept and Prophylaxsis of Childbed Fever (1861), trans. Frank P. Murphy, in Medical Classics, 5 (5-8): 352, Jan.-April, 1941.

24. Frank Gill Slaughter, Immortal Magyar: Semmelweis, Conquerer of Childbed Fever (New York: Schuman, 1950), p. 187.

25. Elizabeth Nihell, A Treatise on the Art of Midwifery (1760) quoted in John Kobler, The Reluctant Surgeon: A Biography of John Hunter (Garden City, N. Y.: Doubleday, 1960), pp. 32-33.

26. Nihell quoted in Kobler, pp. 38-39.

27. Thomas Sydenham quoted by Kenneth Dewhurst, Dr. Thomas Sydenham, 1624-1689: His Life and Original Writings (Berkeley, Calif.: University of California Press, 1966), p. 43.

28. Gideon Harvey quoted by Dewhurst, pp. 43-44.

29. Sydenham quoted by Dewhurst, p. 42.

30. Gaspare Tagliacozzi quoted by Martha (Teach) Gnudi, The Life and Times of Gaspare Tagliacozzi, Surgeon of Balogna, 1545-1599 (New York: H. Reichner, 1950), p. 332.

31. Felix Marti-Ibanez, A Prelude to Medical History (New York: M. D. Publications, 1961), p. 143.

32. Arturo Castiglioni, A History of Medicine, trans. and ed. E. D. Krumbhaar (New York: Knopf, 1947), p. 425.

33. Mrs. Horace Wells, quoted in Betty MacQuitty, Victory Over Pain: Morton's Discovery of Anaesthesia (New York: Taplinger Publ. Co., 1971), pp. 144-145.

34. Horace Wells quoted in MacQuitty, pp. 41-42.

35. Evening Post, Jan. 22, 1848 quoted in MacQuitty, pp. 144-145.

36. Letter from Horace Wells quoted in MacQuitty, pp. 144-145.

37. Almroth Wright quoted in Leonard Colebrook, Almroth Wright, Provocative Doctor and Thinker (London: Heninemann, 1954), pp. 240-1.

BIBLIOGRAPHY

Adams, George Worthington. Doctors in Blue: The Medical History of the Union Army in the Civil War. New York: Henry Schuman, 1952.

Advances in American Medicine: Essays at the Bicentennial. Ed. John Z. Bowers and Elizabeth F. Purcell. New York: Josiah Macy, Jr., Foundation, 1976.

Camp, John Michael Francis. The Healer's Art. New York: Taplinger, 1977.

Cardano, Gerolamo. The Book of My Life. Trans. Jean Stoner. New York: E. P. Dutton & Co., Inc., 1930.

Castiglioni, Arturo. A History of Medicine. Trans. and ed. E. D. Krumbhaar. New York: Knopf, 1947.

Chaplin, Arnold. Medicine in England During the Reign of George III. London: Arnold Chaplin, 1919.

Classics in Psychology. Ed. Thorne Shipley. New York: Philosophical Library, 1961.

Colebrook, Leonard. Almroth Wright, Provocative Doctor and Thinker. London: Heinemann, 1954.

Coulter, Harris L. Divided Legacy, A History of the Schism in Medical Thought. Washington, D. C.: Wehawken Book Co., 1973-77.

Cumston, Charles Greene. An Introduction to the History of Medicine. Rpt. 1926; London: Dawsons, 1968.

Cunningham, Horace Herndon. Field Medical Services at the Battles of Manassas (Bull Run). Athens: University of Georgia Press, 1968.

Dewhurst, Kenneth. Dr. Thomas Sydenham, 1624-1689: His Life and Original Writings. Berkeley: University of California Press, 1966.

The Dictionary of National Biography. Ed. Sir Leslie Stephen and Sir Sidney Lee. London: Oxford University Press, 1917, Vol. VI, pp. 118-120.

Doby, Tibor. Discoverers of Blood Circulation. London: Abelard-Schuman, 1963.

Duffy, John. The Healers: The Rise of the Medical Establishment. New York: McGraw, 1976.

Flack, Isaac Harvey. The Story of Surgery. (Harvey Graham, pseud.) Garden City, N. Y.: Halcyon House, 1943.

Flexner, James Thomas. Doctor on Horseback: Pioneers of American Medicine. New York: Viking Press, 1937.

Forster, John. The Life of Charles Dickens. Rpt. 1927; New York: Everyman's Library, 1966.

400 Years of a Doctor's Life. Ed. George Rosen and Beate Baspari-Rosen. New York: Schuman, 1947.

Garland, Joseph. The Story of Medicine. Boston: Houghton Mifflin Co., 1949.

Glasscheib, Hermann Samuel. The March of Medicine: The Emergence and Triumph of Modern Medicine. Trans. Mervyn Savill. New York: Putnam, 1964.

Gnudi, Martha (Teach). The Life and Times of Gaspare Tagliacozzi: Surgeon of Balogna, 1545-1599. New York: H. Reichner, 1950.

Haggard, Howard Wilcox. Devils, Drugs, and Doctors: The Story of the Science of Healing from Medicine-man to Doctor. New York: Harper & Brothers, 1929.

Johnstone, Robert William. William Smellie: The Master of British Midwifery. Edinburgh: Livingstone, 1952.

Keiffer, John E. "Philadelphia Controversy, 1775-1780." In The Bulletin of the History of Medicine, Vol. 11 (1942), pp. 152-171.

Kobler, John. The Reluctant Surgeon: A Biography of John Hunter. Garden City, N. Y.: Doubleday, 1960.

Lambert, Samuel Waldron and George M. Goodwin. Medical Leaders from Hippocrates to Osler. Indianapolis: The Bobbs-Merrill Co., 1929.

Mackler, Bernard. Philippe Pinel, Unchainer of the Insane. New York: Franklin Watts, 1968.

MacQuitty, Betty. Victory over Pain: Morton's Discovery of Anaesthesia. New York: Taplinger Pub. Co., 1971.

Major, Ralph Herman. The History of Medicine. Springfield, Ill.: Charles C. Thomas, 1954.

Margotta, Roberto. The Story of Medicine. Ed. Paul Lewis. New York: Golden Press, 1967.

Marti-Ibanez, Felix. A Prelude to Medical History. New York: M. D. Publications, 1961.

Maxwell, William Quentin. Lincoln's Fifth Wheel: The Political History of the United States Sanitary Commission. New York: Longmans, Green, 1956.

McKnown, Robin. Pioneers in Mental Health. New York: Dodd, Mead, 1961.

The National Cyclopedia of American Biography. New York: J. T. White and Co., 1899, Vol. 9, p. 259.

Newman, Sir George. Interpreters of Nature. Rpt. 1927; Freeport, N. Y.: Books for Libraries Press, 1968.

Ore, Oystein. Cardano, the Gambling Scholar. Princeton: Princeton University Press, 1953.

Pinel, Philippe. "A Treatise on Insanity." Trans. D. D. Davis Excerpts in Classics in Psychology. Ed. Thorne Shipley. New York: Philosophical Library, 1961, pp. 291-311.

Reconstructive Plastic Surgery: Principles and Procedures in Correction, Reconstruction and Transplantation, 2nd ed. Ed. John Marguis Converse. Philadelphia: W. B. Saunders, 1977.

Riedman, Sarah Regal. Masters of the Scalpel: The Story of Surgery. Chicago: Rand MacNally, 1962.

Roddis, Louis Harry. James Lind: Founder of Nautical Medicine. New York: Schuman, 1950.

Rolleston, Sir Humphry. "The Reception of Harvey's Doctrine of the Circulation of the Blood in England as Exhibited in the Writings of Two Contemporaries." In Essays on the History of Medicine. Ed. Charles Singer and Henry E. Sigerist. Rpt. 1924; Books for Libraries Press, 1968, pp. 247-254.

Rosen, George. 400 Years of a Doctor's Life, coll. and arr. by George Rosen and Beate Caspari-Rosen. New York: Schuman, 1947.

Sabine, Jean Captin. "A History of the Classification of Human Blood Corpuscles." Bulletin of the History of Medicine, Vol. 8, (1940), pp. 696-720.

Semmelweis, Ignaz Philipp. The Cause, Concept and Prophylaxis of Childbed Fever. Trans. Frank P. Murphy. In Medical Classics, Vol. 5, Jan., 1941.

Sigerist, Henry Ernst. The Great Doctors: A Biographical History of Medicine. Trans. Eden and Cedar Paul. New York: Norton, 1933.

Singer, Charles Joseph. A Short History of Medicine. New York: Oxford University Press, 1928.

Slaughter, Frank Gill. Immortal Magyar: Semmelweis, Conquerer of Childbed Fever. New York: Schuman, 1950.

United States Sanitary Commission. The Sanitary Commission of the United States Army: A Succinct Narrative of Its Works and Purposes. Rpt. 1864; New York: Arno Press, 1972.

Venzmer, Gerhard. Five Thousand Years of Medicine. Trans. Marion Koenig. New York: Taplinger, 1968.

Walker, Kenneth, The Story of Medicine. New York: Oxford University Press, 1954.

Walker, M. E. M. Pioneers of Public Health: The Story of Some Benefactors of the Human Race. Rpt. 1930; Freeport, N. Y.: Books for Libraries Press, 1968.

Walsh, Mary Roth. Doctors Wanted: No Women Need Apply: Sexual Barriers in the Medical Profession, 1835-1975. New Haven: Yale University Press, 1977.

Watson, Benjamin P. "How We Learned about the Human Body." In Medicine and Mankind. Ed. New York Academy of Medicine. New York: D. Appleton-Century, 1936.

Watson, Robert Irving. The Great Psychologists: From Aristotle to Freud. Philadelphia: Lippincott, 1963.

Wykes, Alan. Doctor Cardano, Physician Extraordinary. London: Muller, 1969.

Young, Agnes (Brooks). Scalpel: Men Who Made Surgery. (Agatha Young, pseudonym.) New York: Random House, 1956.

Zimmerman, Leo M. "Surgery." In Medicine in Seventeenth Century England: A Symposium Held at UCLA in Honor of C. D. O'Malley. Ed. Allen G. Debus. Berkeley: Berkeley University Press, 1974.

VOLUME III

What lies ahead in Volume III? What compelling vignettes will it contain?

Many readers of Volume I responded to the call for ideas and suggestions. I ask you, the reader of Volume II to do the same. Since Volume III is at least a year away, there is a good amount of time for you to respond. Your suggestions can be of the famous or infamous, just so they changed medical history.

In addition to a third volume of Medical Mavericks, another trilogy is in the planning stages which will be titled Modern Medical Mavericks. By modern I mean those individuals who were born in the 20th Century.

Please send your thoughts as to who should be included in this work as well as Medical Mavericks, Volume III.

Just mail your valued comments to:

Hugh D. Riordan, M.D.
3100 N. Hillside Avenue
Wichita, Kansas 67219 USA

ABOUT THE PUBLISHER

Bio-Communications Press is a service of The Olive W. Garvey Center for the Improvement of Human Functioning, Inc. The Center is a non-profit medical, research and educational organization funded through grants from corporations and foundations and contributions from individuals.

The Center has established three major divisions to carry out its mission of seeking to help stimulate an epidemic of health. These are the ABNA Clinical Research Center, The Bio-Communications Research Institute and The Bio-Medical Synergistics Education Institute.

To learn more about The Center, pictured below, just send your note of request together with a stamped self-addressed #10 envelope to:

The Center
3100 N. Hillside Avenue
Wichita, Kansas 67219 USA

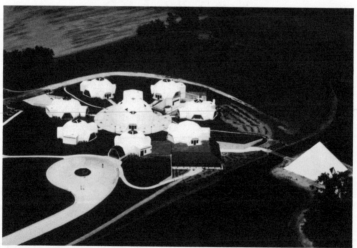

The 21st Century Center Master Facility of 8 geodesic domes and pyramid

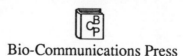

Bio-Communications Press

THERE'S MORE

Bio-Communications Press fulfills a unique niche by publishing fascinating books for select audiences. These books are written by skilled professionals who have demonstrated both a profound interest in their subject matter and the capacity to clearly communicate that interest in an understandable way.

Although our books are not for everyone, we believe what we publish makes a valuable addition to the personal library of anyone who appreciates being well informed on the subject matter they contain.

Our current list of published books:

Medical Mavericks, Volume One–Hugh Riordan, M.D.

The Schizophrenias: Ours to Conquer–Carl Pfeiffer, Ph.D., M.D.

The Vitamin C Controversy: Questions and Answers–
Emanuel Cheraskin, M.D., D.M.D.

The Wonderful World Within You–Roger Williams, Ph.D.

Soon to be released:

Electrodynamic Man–Leonard Ravitz, M.D.

Health and Happiness–Emanuel Cheraskin, M.D., D.M.D.

Hypnosis, Acupuncture & Pain–Maurice Tinterow, M.D., Ph.D.

To receive a list of books currently available from Bio-Communications Press or to be among the first to know when a new book is about to be released, just return the coupon today.

ORDER MORE COPIES

For your friends, colleagues or to donate to your library *Medical Mavericks*, Volumes One and Two are available for only $7.95.

YES!

I want to order _____copies of MEDICAL MAVERICKS, VOLUME ONE

I want to order _____copies of MEDICAL MAVERICKS, VOLUME TWO

NAME _____

ADDRESS _____

CITY _____

STATE _____ ZIP CODE _____

Add $1.50 postage and handling for 1 or 2 books. 3 or more are sent postage paid. Kansas residents add sales tax.

☐ I have enclosed my check for _____

☐ Please charge my credit card

\# |_|_|_|_|_|_|_|_|_|_|_|_|_|_|_|_|_|_|_|_|_|_|

Credit Card: AX___,VISA___,Discover___,MC___

Exp. Date _____

Signature _____

Bio-Communications Press
3100 N. Hillside
Wichita, Kansas 67219 USA

NOTES